Win When You Lose:

A Guide To Successful Dieting

By Susan V. McDaniel

Table of Contents

Preface

This book is for the person who knows what it's like to stand in a clothing store fitting room and have absolutely no piece of clothing look good on their body. It's for the person who tries on the last size they wore and finds it way too small. It's for the person who avoids amusement parks because fitting in the rides' seats is impossible. It's for the person who knows how it feels to turn sideways to fit through a turnstile. It's for the person who always opts for a table at a restaurant rather than a booth because trying to sit at a booth is too uncomfortable.

This book is also for people who have no idea what those situations feel like. People who have never had a weight problem before but gained twenty pounds when they quit smoking can learn how to lose the weight and keep it off, too. Even people who have never before dieted, but now find themselves with a lower metabolism than they have ever had can benefit from this book.

Most "diet books" espouse a certain nutritional eating plan. This one does not. This book instead explains the simple matters of weight control. You'll learn that you must eat food to lose weight. You'll learn how to handle holiday eating. You'll learn that most of us are compulsive overeaters and that's okay. If you aren't a compulsive overeater, you're probably an emotional eater, and that's okay, too. You'll learn how to use the scale to modify behavior; how to judge your success; how to keep from being hungry; how to handle sabotage efforts from friends and family, and strangers too for that matter. And, you'll learn how to maintain the weight loss you've worked so hard to achieve.

The universality of weight loss and weight control transcends any particular weight loss program. All the pitfalls and problems are common to anyone trying to lose weight, no matter what their past experience with weight loss. What it all comes down to is the human factor. There are things you must recognize about psychology, behavior, and physiology. Once you understand these factors, you will be successful at any "diet" you choose to try.

Introduction

You do not have to be "perfect" to lose weight and keep it off. You merely have to be aware, make good food choices more often than not, and be motivated. The premise of this book is that successful weight loss hinges more on psychological issues than what you eat. Everyone knows eating less results in weight loss. The problem is motivating yourself and committing yourself to eating less. Almost any eating plan will work if you work it. But it is very difficult to do that. You get hungry. You don't have time. You seek comfort in food. Who doesn't experience these things? It's how you handle these situations that determines your success or failure. And it's your mindset that gives you the determination to make the changes you need to make. I can help you acquire that winning, successful mindset and ultimately lose weight and keep it off.

Of course, there are people reading this that just want to be told what to eat. This book will help them succeed with whatever eating plan they choose. Any of the many plans available will result in weight loss. But only if you stick with it. You need to know how to cope when your willpower wanes, and that's where this book will help you.

Don't worry. Losing weight does not have to be painful. Losing weight does not have to be difficult. Losing weight does not have to be expensive. Losing weight does not have to be an insurmountable problem. But it is called "dieting", and there's no sugarcoating the fact that you have to diet to lose weight. And dieting presents a conflict.

In fact, it's a war. In the past, the diet wars took no prisoners. You either won or you lost when you dieted…black or white, never grey. Win or lose, never "good try". Only perfection will do. It's pretty simple, and it is also pretty disheartening. Regardless, it's a fight waged over and over again, especially around the first of a new year.

On January 1st, the dieter awakens with a resolve to lose weight unmatched anywhere in the animal kingdom. Those holiday indiscretions, indulgences, and plain old food fests are jiggling around the hips as we walk and sway with each step. With this kind of motivation, the dieter exudes determination and willpower. Unfortunately, this resolve and enthusiasm wanes with each passing hour. By 7 PM on January 1, most people have decided, "What the hell. I've blown it with that 4 PM unscheduled munch-out anyway. And besides, I'm hungry."

All good intentions are given only a passing nod to their previous existence while double portions of New Year's Eve dinner leftovers pass the dieter's lips. Our dieter now becomes KIA - a diet war loser, but not of inches, just of self-esteem.

What people don't understand is that seeing the above scenario as a failure really does doom them to fail before they even get started. Our itinerant dieter has actually succeeded more than failed. More than half of the day has passed with food intake under control. Good choices were made and made consciously. What's the problem with seeing that as a success? But just try suggesting this deviant outlook and the dieter will launch into a tale of food transgression peppered with a huge dose of self-loathing.

"I have absolutely no willpower. I cannot keep from stuffing my face. I'll never lose this weight because I have tried before and never succeeded. This is ridiculous. I will NEVER be thin."

One can try to gently expose the bright side to the dieter's attempt, but again, our past notions tell us dieting is black or white, never gray. Win or lose, never good try. Only perfection will do.

And that's where this book begins. Well, not quite. Usually it takes several weeks before a dieter realizes it is pointless and downright too difficult to go it alone. Only then does the dieter realize the need for a coach, an ally, perhaps a support group.

I have been that coach, that ally, that comforting shoulder for over twenty years: first in a group setting and later in individual sessions. Thousands of dieters have shared their innermost thoughts and feelings with me. Together we have confronted countless obstacles, exposed many myths, devised strategies for success, and shared lots of laughs. Many of the people I counseled have remained lifelong friends and the majority maintained their weight losses.

These tales, anecdotes, and musings have been inspired, sometimes repeated verbatim (although names have been changed to protect the innocent), and fondly remembered from the years I spent helping them become who they wanted to be. Their struggles can help you in your efforts to revamp your eating environment, lose weight, commit to a healthier lifestyle, and be a happier version of you.

Having counseled thousands of people seeking to lose weight and keep it off, I have, as I like to say, "Heard it all and seen it all if not from others, then I've done it myself!" You will see as you read on that I have personally struggled with my own weight my entire life.

There is a commonality between dieters of all ages, backgrounds, sexes, and social status. We are all the same and we all face the same pitfalls and demons. You are not alone, believe me. That realization is a comforting thought to me that I carry around all the time. I share a special bond with all the clients I have known. We have shared struggles and joys, laughter and sadness. We have hugged and cried and known one another well. You have all brought me more happiness and support than you could possibly understand. Now let's go share what we have learned and help someone else

Chapter 1 - Rational Beats Emotional

Are you eating to acquire things food cannot supply? If so, you are an emotional eater and you are not alone. Have you ever exploded in anger at your teenager all the while throwing open the kitchen cabinets to find something (anything!) to eat to make it all okay (and calm you down)? Have you been overwhelmed with a pile of work at the office and so mindlessly devour a bag of M&M's every day at 4 PM? Or how about the stay-at-home mother of little children who finally gets the kids down for an afternoon nap and then runs to the Ben and Jerry's ice cream to savor each spoonful while looking at the clock and wondering how much alone time she has before the little darlings awaken.

Most weight counselors, myself included, advise dieters to separate such emotional situations from food. They would advise, for instance, that in the examples given above the angry parent calmly sit down and express herself rather than turn to food for anger management. The overworked afternoon muncher would be advised to eat more protein at lunch to stave off those afternoon munchies and perhaps to take a walk and ease the stress of so much backlogged work. How taking a walk and leaving the work pile to become even higher relieves stress is one I never fully understood, but I do advise the walk over the M&M's nevertheless. The harried mother would be asked to take a bubble bath rather than indulge in an ice cream orgy. In other words, substitute a positive behavior for stress eating. (There is more about substitution theory later in this chapter.)

Will You Always Be An Emotional Eater? Probably!

All of these suggestions have merit, of course. They all help to remove the emotional aspect of eating and approach stressful situations with a rational attitude. In my mind though, an emotional eater will always be an emotional eater. There is no changing the fact that some of us turn to food for comfort in times of stress. It may shock you to know that not everyone uses food in this way. My husband, my thin husband, simply cannot eat when he is stressed. Food is the farthest thing from his mind in stressful situations. Meanwhile, I'm scanning the horizon for Dunkin' Donuts.

For years I have tried to adhere, personally, to the skinny person creed that says emotional eating must be avoided at all costs in order to maintain a healthy weight. I have failed miserably at all attempts to impart a totally controlled eating response to an emotional situation. Failing to change this aberrant behavior of mine is a source of stress in and of itself.

After years of struggle, I have arrived at three conclusions. First, emotional eating is an ingrained part of my personality. It was probably learned as a child, may even be hereditary in nature, and there simply is no changing the fact that I find comfort from food in stressful situations. Changing that trait would be like trying to change my eye color. I have very dark eyes and even colored contact lenses are useless in changing their hue.

What Can You Do If You Are An Emotional Eater?

The second conclusion I have drawn is that given conclusion number one, I do have control over the types of food I eat in stressful situations. Altering the type of food I eat will also mitigate the damage I do to my waistline during bouts of emotional eating. At such times I usually want the comfort of sweets or carbohydrates. Other people might want salty and crunchy, but my genetic make-up calls for sweets or breadstuffs. Still, I can choose a low-fat frozen yogurt over a premium ice cream, just as I can choose low-fat and low-calorie Italian bread over the real thing. Stressful situations really don't require calorie-laden food. They do sometimes, for some of us, require the action of eating, feeling full, and a dose of feel-good, coping endorphins compliments of carbohydrate metabolism.

Choosing low calorie foods over their fatty counterparts also adheres to the rational over emotional theory because you can just "do the math." Numbers tend to remove the emotional aspect of losing weight and replace it with solid, rational reasoning.

Do The Math

A pound of fat represents 3500 calories. You therefore need to create a 3500 calorie deficit between the amount of energy you take in and the amount of energy you expend to lose one pound. In a week, you would have to have a calorie deficit of 500 calories per day to lose one pound (7 X 500 = 3500). That seems like a lot of deficit to me, which is why I always make it a point to congratulate the person who has "only lost a pound." Losing a pound represents a huge accomplishment in mathematical terms.

That 500-calorie daily deficit is best created half through exercise and half through food intake. Expending 250 calories a day in exercise and taking in 250 fewer calories a day in food will allow you to lose one pound per week. If you can concentrate on this type of rational, mathematical formula in a stressful situation, you are halfway towards taking the emotion out of your weight loss, which is a good thing.

It's also encouraging to recognize that weight loss can come from minor changes in diet as well as major ones. Given the math formula above for calorie expenditure, you could lose 26 pounds in one year by simply replacing two full calorie sodas with diet sodas each day. If you added in a brisk 45 minute walk most days you could increase your weight loss to 52 pounds in a year. How's that for encouraging? Encouraging it may be, but it just doesn't always help in a stressful situation.

How Thinking Like A Thin Person Can Help

The third conclusion discovered about myself is that efforts to change my behavior based on the advice given by most weight loss experts simply doesn't work. Stress saps my energy to the point where I do not want to put on my walking shoes and strut around the neighborhood, even though intellectually (and rationally) I know doing so will make me feel better. Maybe I'm just too old now to have that inner struggle with myself as I try to convince myself that exercise is a great stress reliever. I know it is. I also know that argument does not get me out the door.

The argument that DOES get me out the door is that if I want to be thin, I need to act like thin people act. And thin people address stress through exercise and not through eating. For some strange reason, that thought process works better for me than the "substitution theory" whereby you substitute one behavior for another to reap the same benefits. Call me crazy, but for me, "think thin" works where other thought processes fail.

Another Tactic: Substitution Theory

Other people will get better results with the substitution theory. This entails analyzing what benefit you get from the behavior you wish to change and then finding another way to get the same benefit. You need to think about this plan ahead of time so you have a strategy to deal with the stressful situation before you find yourself mired in it. For instance, let's say you find yourself eating out of loneliness. You are sitting on the couch mindlessly watching television, munching some high-fat food and feeling sorry for yourself. You recognize that you are lonely.

Eating in this situation may make you feel better, but it doesn't address the underlying problem of loneliness. Perhaps a better solution to the situation would be to phone a friend, do some e-mail, or go to an online chat room. All of those solutions will help you feel less lonely and won't add to your weight. Using the computer will keep your hands busy, too, and not with food items.

Another example might be eating out of anger. Many times people suppress their anger by "stuffing their emotions down" with food. Oprah is famous for claiming she does this. Obviously this behavior does not address the real issue of your anger and it adds to your weight problem. Expressing yourself will yield better results.

If you cannot express your anger in words to the person or situation causing your angst, then write down how you feel. Writing your anger down allows you to rationalize your response rather than emotionalize it. It can be most satisfying as a means of expression, too. Writing your feelings may be a one- time answer to a problem or it could become a habit as you create a journal over time. Journaling provides an outlet for your emotions and a safe place to express yourself. It can also take the place of "food solutions" you may have turned to in the past during stressful, anger-filled episodes.

Another likely emotional eating trigger is boredom. Again, you might find yourself on the couch mindlessly munching, just to give yourself something to do. Many people resort to some sort of needlework to ease boredom without food. Keeping your hands busy with crocheting or knitting, or even putting together jigsaw puzzles, is a much better solution to the problem than eating. One friend took up jewelry making and turned it into a successful sideline small business.

A warm bubble bath and a good night's sleep are equally good solutions to the problem of being tired. It's a much better solution than eating. We eat when we are tired to get a temporary boost of energy so we can finish our nighttime chores, or finally get the kids' laundry done, or complete the work we brought home from the office. Likewise, your 4 PM raid on the vending machine at work likely stems from an attempt to avoid an afternoon nap on your office desk.

Substitute, Yes: Replace, No!

Eating when you are tired is an emotional response to a simple problem. You need to get more sleep! Eating does not take the place of sleeping and never will, no matter how much junk food you consume or how many pounds of fat you pack on in an effort to have more energy. Repeat after me: Eating does not replace sleeping.

Lack of sleep is becoming an epidemic in this country. Doctors report an ever- growing number of sleep disorders as police report more and more people are involved in traffic accidents stemming from lack of sleep. While you are not alone in your quest for more energy and more time, if you are eating to acquire things food cannot supply, you are engaging in emotional rather than rational eating. Your weight and your health will suffer accordingly.

H.A.L.T.: Borrow It And Use It

Remember the tenet that many self-help groups use. Never allow yourself to get too Hungry, Angry, Lonely, or Tired. The acronym HALT will help you remember these four deadly emotional traps and help you avoid succumbing to them. Eating will only fix the "hungry" problem, and even at that we know being TOO hungry is a primary cause of overeating.

Things to remember from this chapter:

- Eating does not solve your problems

- A rational approach is great when you can pull it off. Do the math.

- When that fails, at least make "better" choices

- It's OK to be an emotional eater if you devise coping mechanisms

- Think like a thin person

- Try substitution

- Do not eat to acquire things food cannot supply, i.e. sleep, friends.

- Use H.A.L.T.

Chapter 2 - Red Light (Trigger) Foods

It's difficult to admit our own shortcomings.

Take, for instance, the topic of red light, or trigger foods. A green light food is one that we are unlikely to overeat. Think broccoli. Even if you do overeat a green light food, it won't ruin your weight loss efforts. A yellow light food is one that may not appeal to us at another time in another situation, but that we might overeat under certain emotional conditions (anger, loneliness, depression, stress). Think cheese. Too much of a yellow light food and your weight can suffer.

A red light food is one that we are almost always tempted to overeat. For some people the attraction may be the texture (smooth ice cream), for others it would be the taste (salty potato chips), and for others it could be cultural or childhood associations (comforting macaroni and cheese). Excess red light foods will definitely make you gain weight. Everyone generally has about ten foods that can trigger compulsive eating. Overeating of trigger foods is a universal behavior that everyone, even thin people, displays at one time or another.

Deny, Deny, Deny

So imagine my surprise when a friend refused to admit this universal condition. Several people were gathered together, discussing the red light food issue. I noticed Dolores, looking uncomfortable. She fidgeted and tapped her hand on the table until I finally asked, "Are you OK, Dolores?"

"I'm just fine," she retorted. "I just don't have this problem."

Now Dolores was thirty pounds overweight and had yet to fully commit to becoming fit and healthy. I found her denial hard to believe. "Really?" I asked. "Aren't there certain foods you will overeat under certain circumstances?"

"Absolutely not!" she declared with conviction.

She rose to leave and not only did she not address the issue within herself, she also missed one of the funniest discussions I've ever enjoyed.

I started by telling everyone the story of a box of Cocoa Puffs cereal. A friend brought the cereal to me to show a low fat, relatively low calorie food that satisfied her desire for a sweet, chocolate taste. She described how the stuff was so sweet the "sugar comes out your nose." Somehow I ended up taking the entire box of Cocoa Puffs home with me. Unopened, they posed no threat to my eating plan, but the moment I tasted them I was a goner.

I'd eat one cup and fifteen minutes later I'd be back in the kitchen foraging for another cup. Forget that they tasted unbelievably sweet. That was most of the attraction. Another half hour passed and I was back for another cup. By the time the box was three-quarters empty the attitude was that well-worn rationalization, "Well, I just may as well finish them up because I'm going to keep coming back for more until they're all gone anyway."

I related this episode to the friend that gave me the cereal and she looked at me with a thoroughly incredulous expression and snarled, "How could you do that? They're so sweet the sugar comes through your nose." She turned away from me, but cut both eyes back in my direction in a very disdainful gesture.

I was mortified, but also highly amused. I told my friends this sad story and asked them to confess their own red light food indiscretions to make me feel better, and confess they did.

Wendy laughed out loud and scooted to the edge of her chair, her dark brown hair bobbing. She was obviously getting ready to tell a secret. "That's nothing! Cocoa Puffs- bah!" and she shook her head dismissively.

"When I go to the grocery store, I have to stash all the goodies in the extreme back end of my Suburban or else I eat everything before I get home. If I don't put them way back there, I'm reaching over the seat during the whole ride, trying to tell by touch what's what."

She mimicked driving with her left hand on the steering wheel and her right arm flailing behind her as everyone laughed.

"Oh like that isn't an accident waiting to happen!" taunted Ann. "And I thought cell phone talkers were bad."

"Hey, haven't I seen you at the stop lights, Wendy? Wasn't that you getting out and running around to the back of the truck, pawing through the bags, trying to find goodies before the light turns green?" laughed Carla.

I said since our town was so small we could save Wendy from herself when we saw her pulled over on the side of the road, rummaging in her trunk. Now we knew what she was really doing back there, looking for something to eat before she got home. (By the way, at last count, Wendy had lost 75 pounds!)

The spontaneity and honesty Wendy and I shared encouraged other people to talk about their overeating episodes.

"Hey," said Julie, Do you know how fast a pint of ice cream will melt while driving home from Key West?"

"No, but I bet you're going to tell us," we all seemed to say in unison, egging her on.

"Pretty fast unless you get to it by mile marker 5. By then it's melted around the edges and hard in the center," she answered.

"Oh, I love it that way," I interjected.

"Yeah, but if you wait any longer it all turns to mush. Then you refreeze it and it gets ice crystals all through it so you just leave it for the rest of the family! I blame it on the lousy refrigeration system at the grocery store," she laughed.

Everyone roared.

Someone else talked about inhaling a whole tub of movie theatre buttered popcorn and someone else spoke of full bags of potato chips emptied in a flash. It was a cathartic experience to know that everyone falls prey to these behaviors, even people at their goal weights. One lady who is religious about her food intake said someone once told her to freeze Christmas cookies so she wouldn't eat them. She said, "Like that would help! I'd just brush the frost off and eat them frozen. I'm incorrigible."

Deprivation Doesn't Work

The trick with red light or "trigger foods" is to acknowledge our faults and try to minimize their impact. Depriving ourselves of the foods we love is usually not the answer. Deprivation only makes the craving more intense. It may be necessary to keep the food out of reach for a time until eating becomes a more conscious behavior. I've kept peanut butter out of my house for 20-plus years. I'll tell you later about the current status of my relationship with peanut butter. Even so, depriving ourselves of the foods we really love is not the answer to our weight problems.

Enjoying favorite foods in controlled situations is a good alternative. The ice cream served at a restaurant is a controlled portion and probably enough of a treat to keep you satisfied. Similarly, buying favorite foods in a smaller portion, like a snack bag of chips rather than the big bag, may be enough to ward off overeating episodes.

When confronted in your home with red light foods, it's a good idea to divide them into portion controlled increments. Those snack size zip lock bags are perfect for this purpose. Prevent eating the food as it's being divided by chewing gum during the divvying up process, or get someone else to do it for you. Storing these foods out of sight helps, too, because out of sight really is out of mind.

Generally, the temptation to overeat a trigger food is greatest when we have let ourselves get too deprived, too hungry, or too tired. (Remember H.A.L.T. from chapter 1?) Planning well alleviates these trying times and helps make it easier to choose healthy foods. Should you find yourself overindulging, though, remember that you can be out of control one moment and back in control the next if you allow yourself to make that choice.

My own "well I may as well go all the way and finish it up-attitude" is not a foregone conclusion to the situation. It is a choice. Don't make it yours! Instead, take the high road, recognize the damage you are doing, and take some action to end the situation. You'll be glad you did the next time you step on the scale.

Who Caused This Problem? (Or Blame It On Someone Else)

The temptation to overeat a trigger food most often occurs in our own households. The question is then, "How did these foods find their way into our environment in the first place?" The answer is usually that WE BOUGHT THEM. Let me emphasize that we cannot EAT what we do not BUY. What goes into the grocery cart will likely go into our mouths and ultimately ends up on our hips, thighs, and stomachs.

I can't begin to recall how many times parents have argued this indisputable fact with me. The argument usually goes,

"But I have younger children at home."

"So?" I ask.

"I can't deprive them just because I have a problem. They whine in an 'oh so pitiful' voice. Why, that just wouldn't be right."

"Your children can also benefit from eating tasty, nutritious foods. They don't need to eat junk food. It's not good for them, just like it's not good for you."

"But.......But.......I HAVE to buy them chips (or ice cream, or cookies, or whatever)."

It's usually a waste of breath to argue the point. Sometimes parents use the food as a means to control the children and would therefore be wrested of their control without having it in the house; or alternately, the children are merely an excuse to buy the offending products. The parents refuse to admit that the junk food is as much for them as it is for the children.

Children have plenty of access to junk food at their friends' homes and even in some school systems. What they don't have plenty of is good nutritious food and healthy, fit role models. I have seen many children choose grapes over M&M's given the opportunity. Some even prefer raw broccoli rather than potato chips. If we start to teach our children to eat healthy at a young age, the lesson will last a lifetime. Children benefit from having less nutritious foods banned and replaced with fruits and other healthy fare, just as parents benefit.

Our children are experiencing obesity and diabetes at an ever increasing rate at ever younger ages. The statistics from the Center for Disease Control, National Center for Health Statistics say fifteen percent of children ages 6 to 11 are already overweight. The same percentage applies for adolescents aged 12 through 19. However, sixty-four percent of adults over age 20 are overweight, while thirty percent are considered obese. We should not perpetuate obesity and the concomitant illnesses of cancer, diabetes, and heart disease by providing a ready source of junk food in our homes. It makes no sense to provide access to these nutritionally void foods when we are tasked with protecting the welfare of our family.

Furthermore, it makes no sense monetarily to buy trigger foods when money is also being spent for weight control classes, prepackaged foods, gym membership, or a book about diet and nutrition. Wasting money and sabotaging the whole process makes about as much sense as kicking a hornets' nest and complaining when we get stung.

Confess And Deal With It

We must not only be willing to leave these trigger foods in the market, we must also be willing to admit they are trigger foods in the first place. Whenever and wherever I admit this to people they are generally shocked and act totally without understanding to the whole "trigger food behavior." They truly look at me like I have just admitted some horrible sin that should never be spoken aloud.

Recently I was waiting in line at the grocery store and I recognized the lady behind me. She was a memorable character: very outspoken, distinctive appearance, and ready smile. My cart was overflowing with food while hers contained only a few items in the uppermost section. When I noticed her, she was staring intently at a box of reduced-calorie ice cream cones that she had in her cart. The stare was so intense I could almost see her eating them. The treats were a low calorie version of the old-fashioned Nutty Buddy cones - delicious with a capital D. I hadn't bought them in over a year because I knew all too well the effect they have on me. I would eat the entire box in one sitting. They are that good.

I decided to speak to her. "Excuse me…Don't you play tennis at the Sandy Lane courts?" I asked.

"Yes, I do," she responded with that ready smile I had admired the last time I saw her.

"I thought I recognized you. How are you? You look great! Have you lost weight?"

"Thanks. I haven't lost much weight but my clothes fit better from the exercise, I guess," she said. "I'm still trying to lose, though." she said as she reached into her cart and held up the box of ice cream cones.

"Oh, those are so good...."

"I know they are!" she smiled again.

I dropped my voice somewhat, leaned in towards her and said, "But I can't buy those. If I do, I can't eat just one. I'll end up eating the..." I dropped my voice to a whisper, "whole box," and I emphasized 'box.'

She looked like she had just seen and heard a grenade go off next to her. The smile faded, the whites of her eyes appeared, and she abruptly dropped the box of cones into the uppermost section of her cart. With a start, she suddenly began shaking her head and going, "Oh.... No! No!"

I returned to putting my groceries on the conveyor belt, wondering about such an unexpected reaction to my admission. I glanced back and later saw her again looking longingly at the package and gently stroking the edge of the box with one finger in a dreamlike state. It reminded me of someone touching a fine piece of satin material, and daydreaming about what the garment would feel like when worn.

There was no doubt in my mind, that lady would be wearing that entire box of ice cream cones, just like a fine satin gown, the luxury clinging to her hips and swishing about her legs and thighs for a long, long time. The life expectancy of that box of cones was several hours, max. I bet she ate one on her way out of the parking lot! Would she recall what I said and think twice next time she bought them? Maybe. But it would take another conversation for her to realize that she needed to avoid those trigger foods.

Fat Free And Low Carb Is Not Calorie Free Or Low Carb

Just because that food is packaged with a big banner proclaiming it is "Fat Free" or "Low Carb" or "1/3 less calories than the original" or any other deceiving advertising slogan you can think of, does not mean it is inert and will not harm your willpower, your health, and your waistline. Likewise, just because it says "natural" or is produced by a national weight loss company does not necessarily mean it is a good choice and certainly does not mean it can be consumed in unlimited portions.

In fact, some of those reduced-fat, reduced-calorie foods are the most likely to be overeaten because they are the least satisfying. Removing the fat (and oftentimes replacing it with sugar or sugar substitutes) tends to make them very unfulfilling. This phenomenon explains why a small full-fat ice cream would satisfy your craving better than the whole box of fat-free ice cream cones.

Desensitization To Trigger Foods

I do, however, want to give you hope that in time you can learn to deal with the foods you find so tempting. In psychology circles there is a behavior modification technique known as "desensitization." This process is usually used for people with phobias. An example might be someone with a fear of thunderstorms. The first step in the desensitization process would be to listen to a tape or CD of a storm. Then you would progress to viewing one from a long distance. Then you might sit in your car during a storm. The idea is to slowly become accustomed to the thing that frightens you until it is no longer a threat.

The same process can happen with red-light foods. It happened to me. Peanut butter has been a red-light food for me since I was pregnant with my son 29 years ago. Up until that time, I never ate it and actually detested it. For some reason, it became delectable to me during pregnancy. It has remained delectable for 27 years. It is so delectable that I cannot control my consumption to a mere serving. Instead, I have to eat the whole jar, no matter what size that jar might be.

Purely by accident, I ended up going through the desensitization process. It happened when my dog needed handfuls of medication each day and I had to find a vehicle for the medications that he would eat. I had been using a particular dog food but he suddenly developed a dislike for it. (Probably because it was stuffed with pills!) Someone suggested peanut butter and I thought, "No way am I having peanut butter in my house! I'll eat it myself and blow up like a balloon!"

Naturally, the dog's needs come before my own because that's how it is when you love a dog (or two). Peanut butter ended up on my kitchen counter and I began using it three times a day to feed my dog his medications. At first the smell and texture were overpowering. I ate several slices of warm toast smothered in peanut butter. I also noticed that I wasn't hungry for hours afterwards. (That's always a clue that I've eaten what I shouldn't have eaten!)

As days wore on, I found that I could give Buster his medication without licking the spoon. I also found that I didn't want to eat a spoonful myself. I found that I still enjoyed the smell but it wasn't causing me to salivate anymore. The desensitization process seems to have worked for my peanut butter compulsion. The jar is now in the kitchen cabinet. I can't assure you I won't devour it in the future given the right (or wrong) mental attitude and circumstance, but for the moment, the compulsion is under control.

In the first stages of a weight loss journey, it is easiest to simply ban any trigger foods from your environment until you lose the weight you need to lose. But after that, test the waters and see what reaction the trigger foods cause. Just bear in mind that it took me 20+ years to allow the Jif Bunny to reside in my house. It may take just as long for you to live comfortably with Little Debbie.

Do Not Eat Food You Don't Like

After banning your favorite foods, do not make yourself eat foods you do not like in the name of "dieting." During past diet attempts I ate mountains of cottage cheese and tuna. Didn't we all? I still eat them at times but they evoke memories of past diet failures. I do not force myself to eat them to lose weight anymore. Since your intake of food is being limited, you should only eat the foods you really love. Old foods deemed diet foods tend to make us feel more deprived than we should. There's a connotation of dieting and deprivation there that we need to avoid.

Likewise some packaged foods are less than tasty. I vividly recall a prepackaged meal of yesteryear called "Spaghetti Bolognese." I tried to eat this frozen meal while the rest of my family ate real homemade spaghetti. It was so awful (it had square "meat bits," for heaven's sake!) I finally gave up trying to eat it. In fact, I ended up giving it to our very expressive dog. She took one bite of a "meat bit" and turned her head from side to side in a quizzical way as if to ask, "What the heck are you trying to feed me?????" The moral is, save your food allotment for foods you enjoy and don't force yourself to eat things your dog finds questionable.

Trigger foods certainly contribute to our weight struggles and cause us to overeat at times. However, even without a particularly delectable food, compulsive overeating remains a hurdle for all of us to overcome. We can limit our exposure to red light foods that trigger us to overeat, but our inherent desire to overeat compulsively remains a problem we must face.

Red Light (Trigger) Foods

Things to remember from this chapter:

- Everyone has trigger foods that they will overeat under certain circumstances.

- Empower yourself by getting rid of foods you may compulsively overeat. Then do not buy any more trigger foods. You cannot eat what you do not buy.

- Do not deprive yourself of the foods you love. Plan to eat them in controlled portions in controlled settings, at least. Have dessert in a restaurant or splurge on a snack sized bag of potato chips once in a while.

- If the offending food must be in your home, keep it out of sight and in metered portions.

- Children and "non-dieting" family members also benefit from having only nutritious food in the house. Eating well is not a punishment.

- Important: Low-fat foods can be just as damaging as other foods when eaten in large quantities. Do not be hoodwinked into thinking you can eat unlimited amounts of these foods. Many times these are major trigger foods because they are the least satisfying.

Chapter 3 – The Compulsion To Overeat

Banning red light foods from the environment helps control the tendency to overeat. Particular foods aside, however, most people with long-standing weight problems are compulsive overeaters, independent of red light or trigger foods. If you give us an inch, we'll take a mile.

In fact, we are all compulsive overeaters given the right circumstance and the right food. Information, moderation, damage control, removing temptation, and recognizing our tendencies are the best coping mechanisms we can hope to achieve.

If It Sounds Too Good To Be True ....

In the spring of 2001 a product became all the rage in the area where I worked and lived. News flew around the world via the internet that this low fat ice cream was a 12-ounce single serving for a mere 150 calories. The brand name was Big Daddy Ice Cream produced by the DeConna Ice Cream Company of Orange Lake, Florida. People even organized letter-writing campaigns to have this product made available at their local grocery stores.

The product was amazingly popular in dieting circles. Twelve ounces of almost anything for just 150 calories is cause for excitement! I'm not saying we were consuming the stuff in unlimited quantities, but we were eating more that we should have been. And it really did taste like a low fat ice- milk type product. It wasn't all that tasty. In fact, it seemed like it could have had "quintessionally frozen product" on the label like some of the other ice pop products.

On June 17, 2001 reporter Mitch Lipkin wrote an expose for the South Florida Sun Sentinel newspaper. Mr. Lipkin apparently knew when something was too good to be true even if we didn't. He had a container of the Big Daddy Ice

Cream analyzed and found that a 12-ounce serving contained not 150 calories but 300! It also had 7.5 grams of fat and 50 grams of carbohydrate. No wonder we weren't losing weight like we should have been!

When dieters heard the news they were appalled. One normally mild-mannered woman was livid. "They should all be killed," she growled, and I think she meant it. Another said, "Fraud. Pure fraud. They exploited us and they knew just what they were doing." She almost spit in the dust after her last word. It's possible the manufacturer knew exactly what it was doing. Who knows? But shouldn't we have known that we were overindulging?

We did know. But we're always looking for that delicious food that we can eat to our heart's content without it showing on our hips. Unfortunately, that food doesn't exist and companies prey on us because they know we are looking for it.

Way Too Much Of A Good Thing

Another example of this compulsive behavior involved a product called "Breakfast Cookies." They contained an enormous amount of fiber so they seemed like a good choice and a low fat/low calorie food. The company that made them obviously knew they were manipulating the system for their own benefit but again, we were taken in. The company demanded that an order contain several dozen cookies so friends pooled individual orders. A week later UPS delivered a sixty-pound box of cookies to my doorstep. In retrospect, there was something very, very wrong with that scenario.

Just one of the cookies weighed half a pound and was delicious. People used them as cereal substitutes for breakfast but overeater that I am, I could not eat just one. Even freezing them didn't help. I just brushed off the frost along the edges and popped them in the microwave to defrost. Microwaving actually improved the taste. (It's a good thing I don't have access to my friend's Christmas cookies from the last chapter!)

Recognizing the temptation to overeat them, I dropped out of the bulk mailing group but others continued to order and consume these monsters. High fiber does not mean low calorie. I think we're all lost causes sometimes.

Don't Believe Everything You Read

Recently, the Nutrition Action Newsletter, a publication of the nutrition watchdog group, Science in the Public Interest, revealed similar labeling defects by manufacturers. This information appeared in the June, 2003 issue in an editorial memo from Dr. Michael Jacobson. Highlighted were two prominent examples of "fakers in the food aisles." One was the McDonald's low-fat ice cream cone. Everyone loves this treat because it is supposedly only 150 calories, according to information supplied by McDonald's.

The problem is the serving size noted is three ounces (90 grams). Those three ounces are the serving size for which McDonalds provides calorie and fat information. The treat, however, is routinely 135 grams as purchased: a fifty percent increase over the stated serving size, so the calorie and fat counts are proportionately larger. In fact, the average of those cones purchased by the Center for Science in the Public Interest contained 225 calories. Apparently, a three- ounce cone would be one filled only to the brim of the cone itself. Now when was the last time you saw an ice cream cone served that way? Recalling the way in which these cones are filled may help you understand that each server adds a different amount of ice cream to each cone.

And thank you also for noting that the premium beef in the grocery store known as Laura's Beef, while free of hormones and other additives, is not as low-fat as the label portends. Their rib eye steaks have recently been stripped of the heart healthy, low fat labels they used to sport because the fat content was analyzed and found to be too high. Center for Science in the Public Interest purchased ribeye and strip steaks at random, analyzed them, and reported that each contained an average of 40 percent more calories than the label stated. (Saturated fat was twice what the label reported.)

Laura's strip steaks have been granted permission to sport the American Heart Association (AHA) "heart check" on their labels but only one of the strip steaks analyzed met the AHA's criteria. The Center reports that two steaks had three times the limit of saturated fat. The AHA has since removed their logo from the ribeye steaks and we assume that they will similarly yank them off of the strip steaks after widespread publication of this report. Laura's certainly makes a wonderful product, however. It is tasty, relatively healthy for beef, and I'm sure they will rectify the labeling problems.

Similarly, the July/August 2003 issue of Weight Watchers magazine notes that a popular snack called Pirate's Booty and Veggie Booty was recalled by the Federal Drug Administration last year. According to the article, the cheese and veggie-flavored corn snacks were marketed as containing 120 calories and 2.5 grams of fat per serving. Well, that was a little understated.

The Good Housekeeping Institute analyzed the snacks and found that a one-ounce serving, less than a snack bag, tipped the scales at 147 calories and 8.5 grams of fat. The snacks now carry the correct nutritional information but how many people ate them and wondered why the pounds weren't dropping off? Of course, if we weren't overeating them, the discrepancy probably wouldn't have had much effect on our weight loss.

The Weight Watcher article advises that most nutrition labels can be trusted and my examples are the exceptions to the rule. We must be especially careful to note the serving size that the information is calculated upon, however. Also, we are advised to note that the government does not monitor nutritional information for products sold at the corner deli, coffeehouses, or ice cream parlors. That's why the big old cranberry-orange muffin that is labeled "low fat" keeps us from being hungry for seven hours. The chances of it truly being low-fat are low odds.

We rely heavily on nutrition labels to make informed decisions about which food to purchase and consume especially when we're trying to lose weight. We need to recognize that labels are not infallible. They are sometimes used unscrupulously as marketing tools by manufacturers rather than as simply reliable consumer information.

We know that eating a rib eye steak is consuming a lot of fat and calories, label or no label. We're also smart enough to know that a McDonald's cone really is more satisfying than some other snacks. That's why we keep going back for more! In essence, we are smart and aware enough to know when something is too good to be true, whether we admit it or not. It is just our nature to take advantage of such situations, fool ourselves into thinking our over-consumption is okay, and wonder why we aren't losing any weight.

While it is justified to hold food manufacturers to strict standards when it comes to supplying nutritional information, we must bear personal responsibility for our food intake. No one is holding a fork to our mouth except us. No one but us is responsible for what we put into our "pie hole." We all know when we are being compulsive and we are responsible for the consequences. Moderation is the magic word.

Compulsion And Sabotage

Sharon is a lovely lady, 50-something, who gained weight after her husband died unexpectedly. She managed to lose the weight and actually lost too much. I was concerned for her health and suggested on more than one occasion that she was dangerously close to being anorexic. She denied it, of course. Only several years later did she tell me, "I just stopped eating."

Sharon ended up moving and got away from dieting entirely. She gained back all the weight she had lost. The last time I spoke to her she was lamenting the fact that she was all alone, wasn't cooking or eating healthfully, in fact, she was almost powerless against her own compulsions.

"I ate a whole jar of peanut butter last night. Then I started on crackers and cheese. I just can't help myself," she moans.

I remain quiet, not advising, just listening when she adds, "A few weeks ago a friend took me to Wal-Mart and they had the most delicious little bite sized éclairs in a tub with 75 of them. Mmmmmm. I ate the whole thing in 24 hours."

Now I'm wondering why she is telling me this and if it's to tempt me or to soothe her own soul. "Why would you do such a thing?" I ask.

"I don't know," she sighs. "They were so good."

Several weeks later she relates almost the exact same story only this time she and her friend ate the éclairs right out of the tub on the car ride home from the store.

"So you bought them again? You know you are being compulsive so stop sabotaging yourself and stop buying them," I admonished her with my best motherly voice.

"I know I shouldn't but I just can't help myself."

I feel bad for Sharon because I know how hard she worked to lose the weight in the first place but there's nothing I can do to help her until she helps herself. No one is buying this junk food for her except her. It is her responsibility to put a stop to such bad behavior. I thoroughly understand her problem (see Dulce de Leche below) but there comes a time when we can no longer moan and groan about a situation of our own making.

Sharon and I are good examples of compulsive overeaters. I doubt she would admit to the label, but it fits perfectly. Not many people I have known allow themselves to be categorized like that, but our behavior reveals the truth.

Potluck

At various times I've organized potlucks to introduce people to low-fat cooking. Everything must be low- fat, healthful food with the recipe and nutritional information attached. The idea behind these festivities is that boredom with the food we eat while trying to lose weight is a major cause of failure. Many times eating the same foods day in and day out will get you the weight loss you're looking for, but the cost of doing this in terms of eating satisfaction is too dear. The only way to embrace the healthy eating plan as a way of life is to make it tasty and enjoyable.

The last time we had a potluck we had some really fabulous dishes appear. Lots of them were entirely original but some were prepared products right out of the box and others were recipes gleaned from the annals of helpful publications like Cooking Light and Health magazines. I intended to set up the food on tables provided and to perform an introductory lecture about healthy cooking methods.

Unfortunately, I couldn't get the people away from the food! They positioned themselves like vultures around the food tables, gabbing and chatting and nibbling before the starter's pistol even sounded. I should have known combining people with weight issues and an abundance of food would be a problem.

All in all, the idea was a success. Everyone left with new ideas and new recipes to try and they went away motivated to replace unhealthy fare on their dinner tables with "better choices." The only one that went away hungry was me. I got involved chatting while everyone else was noshing. By the time I ventured over to the food tables, plates of crumbs were the only evidence that a great potluck dinner had been served. Note for future potlucks: Get my plate of food first!

I laughed at them all, "You all were like vacuum cleaners around this food! It's no wonder we all have weight problems! Good grief. Where did all that food go?"

A smart aleck young lady named Diane quipped, "Well, we left the recipes for you!"

Admit It And Deal With It

Every overweight person must realize, admit, and understand that their relationship with food is the result of years of conditioning, learning, and repetition of behavior. This relationship isn't likely to change in a heartbeat so it's better, in my opinion, to acknowledge that we love to eat and find healthy ways of doing just that. Ignoring or denying that we are, or can be under certain circumstances, compulsive overeaters does not alleviate the problem or get us any closer to our weight loss goals.

Some people expect that once they join a weight loss program or decide to lose weight, they will magically be transformed into people who couldn't care less about food. Why this is a common misunderstanding is really beyond my comprehension. Perhaps some weight loss plans do expect unconditional adherence to "the plan," but that is a naïve expectation. Not allowing for transgressions and indiscretions results in people who complain about "cheating" and "feeling guilty." Guilt only makes us want to eat more. It is not an emotion conducive to weight loss and management.

The Compulsion To Overeat

I always try to convince people that overeating is not the sin they have always believed it to be. Years of conditioning and mind washing have us believing that overeating is shameful. But the truth is that everyone, even thin people, overeats at one time or another. The event is not the issue; what happens after the event is what is important.

The following story reveals that overeating is common to everyone struggling with weight management, and that includes people at their weight goals. I went to the grocery store looking for a new product called Silhouettes Ice Cream Sandwiches. These were considered "legal goodies" because they were low in fat and calories. I hunted for several weeks and finally complained to a friend of my frustration in not being able to locate these goodies. It turns out that most everyone I knew confessed to hoarding the darned things. People actually staged a lookout that notified everyone in town by cell phone when the goodies were discovered at a particular store.

Nell, a perfectly quaffed, always dignified and not-a-hair-out-of-place 75 year-old said, "Well Susan, I suppose if you desire a box of those ice cream treats that much I could let you have one of mine. I recently purchased several boxes and have them stored in my freezer."

"Several boxes?" I inquired. As she smiled her perfectly composed little smile, her head tilted ever so slightly, "Yes, I said 'several'."

"And how many exactly is 'several,' Nell?" I doggedly continued.

A faint little voice said, "Nine."

"NINE? NINE?" I erupted. "Nell, nine is totally over the top and unacceptable. No more hoarding these things and definitely no more binging on them, OK?"

Again, the faint little voice, "But they're so hard to get."

"They're hard to get because you all are hoarding them," I replied.

Having finally located and purchased these goodies, I understood the compulsion to stockpile them. They were addictive. The problem was they simply did not satisfy. They were virtually fat-free and sweetened with artificial sweetener, so rather than quell our appetite they instead made us want to eat more than we should. This phenomenon was mentioned in the previous chapter. It is a trait of many trigger foods. They are not satisfying.

Many fat free foods have this effect. People tell me specifically that they have a hard time controlling their consumption of Snack Well cookies and crackers. One serving turns into the whole box in the blink of an eye. This problem doesn't occur because we are "bad" people or because we are "out of control." This problem occurs because of the constituents of the food. Low-fat, sugar-laden food simply makes us hungry for more, rather than satisfy our craving. Could these foods be designed for that purpose? It makes you wonder, doesn't it?

Anyway, I went looking for a substitute yummy when I couldn't locate the Silhouettes Ice Cream Sandwiches and ended up discovering the wonders of Healthy Choice Dulce de Leche Low-Fat Ice Cream. This product has only 120 calories, or thereabouts, per 1/2 cup and for that reason it made its way into my shopping cart. Besides, I'd never been a real ice cream fan and it never dawned on me that this food would pose a challenge of any sort. I had never tasted "Dulce de Leche"-anything before so I really didn't know what it was except that it is very popular in our community because of the Cuban influence on our cuisine.

It turned out to be low-fat caramel ice cream with ribbons of caramel throughout. It was absolutely scrumptious and I couldn't resist it. I inhaled the first half-gallon. (Note: Do not ever be lulled into thinking that a low-fat food can be consumed in unlimited quantities. Many low-fat foods have just as many calories as regular foods because manufacturers replace the fat with extra sugar.) The ribbons of caramel had particular appeal. I dug those out and ate them right off the spoon!

On my next trip to the grocery store I strode right past the frozen foods and didn't even look into the ice cream section. I got home, unloaded the groceries, and lo and behold, what are the odds? Someone had placed that very same ice cream into my cart! I can only assume the "someone" was me.

I stared at that new half-gallon and thought, "I can either eat this or apply it directly to my butt and hips." In a moment of untold strength and fortitude I realized that this was a new trigger food for me and I had to get rid of it, pronto. After all, one of my steadfast rules is do not have trigger foods available at my home (or yours, either).

It pained me, but I began scooping the ice cream into the sink. Watching it melt was heart wrenching, but it really wasn't melting fast enough. I was afraid I'd eat it right out of the sink if it didn't hurry up and melt. I used the sprayer and squirted water on it. The spray created ridges of ice cream with rivulets of melting cream and water. It helped to see it slip down the drain faster than the melting process alone. However, scooping it into the sink became more and more difficult as I got closer to the bottom of the container. Soon I was eating the caramel ribbons before the stuff was hitting the mound in the sink. I figured I was entitled to the caramel, at the very least, since I was being so virtuous.

Then, I swear, honestly, that mound of melting ice cream screamed, "SAVE ME! I'm melting!" I grabbed the spoon and thought, "Hang on! I'll save you..." and then I pictured how pathetic it would look for me to be eating that stuff out of the sink. I admit I took one spoonful, but then sanity reigned.

Finally, I managed to get rid of the whole container and felt a degree of power when I threw the container in the trash. I never again purchased that particular product knowing the control it had over me. Funny, too, because ice cream is really not one of my favored foods. I don't profess to be perfect. Far, far from it! But you don't have to be perfect to stay at a healthy weight.

My reaction to the overeating, however, resulted from years of experience. Throwing out a food we love is a learned reaction. It is not a natural one. Experience teaches that we can be out of control one minute and back in control the very next, if we choose to be. Usually the reaction to overeating is different. The thought pattern usually goes something like, "Well, I've blown the whole day now that I ate that pizza (doughnut, cake, cheese, peanut butter, etc., etc. Choose one or more.) and so I may as well just eat whatever I want for the rest of the day and start over tomorrow (or next week, or Monday, or after vacation, etc., etc. Choose one or more.)"

Sound familiar? Of course it does. It's a natural reaction to feeling deprived of the foods we love. One slip-up becomes a convenient excuse for us to indulge in whatever we've been missing and craving.

Carol lost 25 pounds and was well on her way to her 35-pound goal when the windy weather broke and a perfect boating day arrived. "I was so excited to be out on the water again. I thought I could swim and snorkel and enjoy getting the exercise I needed," she said with a smile. "I didn't expect it to be a test of my determination to lose those last ten pounds, and certainly not a test that I would fail miserably."

"I went to the grocery store and got a veggie sub for myself and an Italian sub for my husband. I picked up some fruit while he went to get some beer. It never occurred to me that he would buy a huge bag of potato chips, too! In fact, I never saw them until we were way out fishing. I thought, 'I can just have a handful and they won't hurt me.' The handful turned into most of the bag. I was just so unprepared for the situation, but I won't be unprepared again," she declared. "It wouldn't have been a big problem if he had bought two snack size bags, but a huge one was too much temptation. I just couldn't control myself."

"So did your husband make it back to port or did you arrive solo?" I joked.

Natural reactions like Carol's just compound our compulsive overeating tendencies. She had resisted her favorite foods for so long that she was caught short when confronted with a large quantity unexpectedly, without a contingency plan of action. That's why we have to have a plan when disaster strikes and we find ourselves out of control. How can we get back on track without letting one slip turn into a week long slide? The answer is different for everyone but some suggestions include:

- Exercise (take a walk) to distract yourself from the temptation or situation causing you to overeat.

- Examine the situation, especially the emotions involved, so you can learn what triggered the overeating and avoid it in the future.

- Plan your next meal, or meals for the rest of the day. I don't mean that you should starve to compensate for what you overate. You should go right back to a healthy eating plan. You can try to compensate through exercise but don't overdo that either! Binging and starving or binging and over-exercising is not the way to a healthy weight. They may be natural reactions, but we've seen what effect those can have.

- I must repeat myself: Low-fat foods can be just as damaging as other foods when eaten in large quantities. Do not be hoodwinked into believing you can eat unlimited amounts of these foods.

- Talk to a friend, e-mail someone, write a blog, check out an online support group. Stop by the "Win When You Lose" Facebook page and share your thoughts. Visit at http://www.facebook.com/WinWhenYouLose

- Don't ever let yourself get too hungry because that's when it's most difficult to control your food intake. Plan ahead and snack often to avoid this situation.

Hunger Breeds Compulsive Overeating

As a final note, let me illustrate how destructive it can be to allow yourself to become too hungry. One day in my late teens I had worked two jobs and was heading to a third when a friend asked me to have dinner with him. He suggested a legendary steakhouse in downtown Baltimore. I had never been there before, and since he was paying, I agreed to dine with him. The restaurant was called The House of Welsh.

I had not eaten one morsel of food all day long. No breakfast, no lunch, no snacks, nothing. When I entered the House of Welsh at 5:30 PM I was famished, and dehydrated, too, probably. The signature dish at this place was a sizzling Porterhouse steak that weighed 24 ounces. It was served on a sizzling platter, and the challenge was that if you could finish one, they would give you another one for free.

Do I even need to tell you who polished off two of these monsters? My companion was thoroughly pleased to have me meet the challenge and at the moment, I was, too. The whole restaurant stared as the management made a spectacle of honoring their promotional challenge by presenting me with yet another sizzling steak, toted high above the waiter's head on a sizzling platter. After much pomp and circumstance, the new steak was planted firmly in front of me. I ate that one, too.

Twenty-four ounces of steak times two equals 48 ounces. With sixteen ounces in a pound, that amounts to three pounds of steak. Even if we disallow the bone and trimmings, that's a lot of meat. As I recall there was also a salad and French Fries as accompaniments. That memorable meal occurred 35 years ago, but it could just as easily happen tonight. Happily, I now understand that starvation dieting always backfires, and being overly hungry leads to compulsive overeating.

We are all compulsive overeaters given the right circumstance and the right food. Damage control, removing temptation, and recognizing our tendencies are the best coping mechanisms we can hope to achieve.

Things to remember from this chapter:

- Everyone is a compulsive overeater given the right food and circumstance.

- Moderation is the key. You cannot compulsively overeat. Not even foods deemed "low fat" or "low calorie" can be eaten with wild abandon.

- Do not believe every nutrition label you read, and watch for serving size on the labels.

- You can be out of control one minute and back in control the next.

- Do not let yourself get too hungry or you will set yourself up for overeating.

Chapter 4 - Sabotage: Don't Let Them See You Sweat

One of the most disheartening things that can happen to a person trying to lose and or maintain their weight is to encounter a saboteur. The episode may truly undermine the self-esteem of the dieter, no matter who they are or how long they've been working at the weight loss or maintenance process. Sabotage comes from people you know and trust, when you least expect it, which makes it particularly damaging.

Frenemy Sabotage

For example, I had been at my goal weight for almost nine years having lost a total of 45 pounds over an initial ten-month period. I was a seasoned weight loss counselor, knowledgeable, and successful in maintaining my weight. None of that experience insulated me from the effects of the sabotage with which I was often confronted. In fact, I think my job as a counselor actually made me a target for a lot of people.

One of the most vivid episodes involved a "friend" whom I eventually helped to lose thirty pounds. She and I were an unlikely duo, but we struck up a friendship, nonetheless. She was older, heavier, and an outspoken funny lady. She was not successful in her initial weight loss attempt and months passed before she found her way back to me. During her second attempt, we took a liking to one another. We kept abreast of the events in each other's lives, through notes and phone calls, even when she returned north for the summer months. I thought of her as a staunch ally and compassionate ear in my struggle to maintain my weight loss.

At one point I told some people about a dress I had bought the week before. I went to a local resort that was having a "summer clearance sale," which is the only way I could afford to buy anything at this particular dress shop. As it happened, a neighbor worked at the gift shop there and had told me about some dresses that were on sale. Always looking for affordable dresses to wear to work, I checked it out.

The dresses were a stretchy, crinkle type material popular in the tropics because of their light weight and breathability. The crinkle material also alleviates the need to iron and doesn't look wrinkled even in our high humidity. Being alone with my neighbor in the store at the time, she advised me to simply stretch the dress to fit. So I took it into the dressing room.

I stretched and I stretched and I wiggled and tugged. No matter what the gyration, I could not stretch the dress enough for it to do anything except stick to me like glue. Every ripple and bulge showed. The dress seemed like a sausage casing to me so I threw open the dressing room door and loudly stated, "I look like a sausage!!"

The recently empty gift shop just happened to suddenly be full of people who turned to look at the "sausage lady" in the red dress as I sheepishly withdrew backwards into the dressing room and quietly drew the curtain closed in embarrassment. I peeked out a time or two before finally exiting the dressing room sometime later. My neighbor assured me the dress would stretch once I washed it. Taking her at her word, I bought the dress.

I told this story the following week and everyone encouraged me to wear the dress, which I did sometime later. I can't say for sure if my friend heard the story behind the dress or not, but she was there when I wore it.

I wore the dress, and true to my salesperson friend's word, it had stretched into a nice flirty skirt with a figure hugging bodice. I knew that it may have also hugged my hips a little too tightly and that you could see a bulge or two that shouldn't have been revealed but hey, I'm not 22 years old anymore, and I don't expect perfection. I liked the color and I felt good in the dress. I was feeling pretty perky when my friend approached.

"Sue, there are some articles of clothing certain people should never wear and for you it's that dress. It just doesn't flatter you and you should never wear it again," she stated quite succinctly as she turned on her heel and walked away.

I was dumbfounded. My mouth gaped open. But nothing came out.

I was speechless.

I was insulted.

I was grateful for her candor and embarrassed that I had just stood in front of all of those people looking so unattractive. Believing her to be my friend and believing her to have my best interests at heart, I never wore that dress again. I see it every time I go into my closet and I try it on but the bulges are still there. I haven't yet had the liposuction I apparently need to wear it again.

A year and a half passes and I remain friends with this lady, though at arm's length. During that time she keeps telling me about a dress she has that she wants me to try on.

"It's an expensive dress. I'd like you to have it. I'll bring it to you next time we see each other," she tells me over and over again.

Finally we do see each other and she tells me she has the dress in her car. I go with her to retrieve it. It is in a plastic bag and I take it gratefully and give her a big hug and kiss for thinking of me. I really do appreciate the gesture and I'm looking forward to having something new to wear.

"Now, I had this dress taken in at one time so there should be enough material there for you to let it out if you need to," she says.

That comment made no sense to me since she was always much larger than I, but I let it pass without saying anything. I thought perhaps she meant I could have it made longer since she was very short and I am on the tall side.

"OK. Thank you so much, Jane. It's so sweet of you to think of me. I'm sure it'll be fine. I'll let you know how it fits when I get a chance to try it on."

Hours later I remove the dress from the bag. A multitude of material slips out of the bag. There's so much material there that it actually feels heavy in my hands. A beige twill tent of a dress emerges. The vastness of it makes my mouth drop. As I hold it by the shoulders I notice pretty embroidery of an elephant and a giraffe on the bodice, which is dwarfed by the immenseness of the dress itself. I look for a tag with a size on it and find none. It has to be at least a size 2X. I wear a 12, sometimes a 10, and on a rare occasion when something is mismarked, an 8.

I stand there with this dress staring at me and ask myself, "Does Jane really think I could wear this? Oh my God, how huge do I really appear to everyone? The outside world thinks I'm this big? I am trying to counsel them to lose weight and what do they see? "

My self-confidence was severely shaken. I showed the dress to my husband and he couldn't understand why she had given it to me, either. Weeks passed before I saw her again and she inquired, "So how was the dress?"

Without thinking about it I blurted out, "It was huge on me."

Sabotage: Don't Let Them See You Sweat

You know what she said? She said, "Oh well congratulations. I'm glad," as though I had done something tremendous to make it not fit.

The whole episode seemed like a perfect example of sabotage so I told the entire story to my clients the next week. I even put the dress on over what I was wearing to illustrate how big it was on me. Audible gasps rose from the audience.

The gasps were followed by people saying, "She's your friend?" "No, she's not your friend!" "She's jealous of you." "If you don't wear that red dress again she wins." "You should wear that dress the next time you see her." "No, you should wear the red dress under that dress the next time you see her!" "You should never be alone with this person again. See her only in a group setting." "You should tell her exactly how big that is on you." And then,

"I have a friend who did the same thing to me. She owns a dress shop and she told me she had the perfect dress for me. She showed it to me and it was a 1X and I had already lost 20 pounds!" This story comes from a small, petite lady who barely weighs 100 pounds .Is it any wonder she has trouble recognizing how thin she really is?

"What happened?" I ask.

"I felt like, 'Oh my. Is this how the world sees me? How big does she think I am? I need to lose a lot more weight if she thinks I'm this big.'"

"I felt exactly the same way! But you see that it wasn't real, right? It was just an act of sabotage. The thing about sabotage is you never know from where or when it's coming and that makes it more difficult to deal with because we are at ease and feel safe with the saboteur. We're caught unaware when the person we think is our friend turns on us."

Silent Sabotage

Another friend related her experience when she returned "home" after losing thirty pounds.

"I walked into the neighborhood bar where "everyone knows your name." People hadn't seen me since I'd lost weight so everyone was saying how great I looked and remarking over how different I looked. One guy even said, 'You look like a million bucks!' So I found my friend who was in the back. She has told people that I'm her best friend but I don't feel that way about her. She's my friend but we aren't that close. Even so, I sat down next to her and told her how great she looked because she did. She always looks smart and put together.

"She never said a word to me. Sitting next to her was her sister, so her sister elbowed her and said, 'Look how much weight she's lost! Doesn't Jean look great?' My friend said, 'Yeah. I noticed her arms are a little smaller.'"

I asked, "So how did that make you feel?"

"Oh, I was mad but I figured she was just jealous. She's not my best friend."

Many times silence is the greatest sabotage. One lady that had lost 30 pounds went home for the holidays expecting a wonderful response from her family and friends who had not seen her at her new, healthy weight.

I was excited for her and rushed up to her after New Year's. "Tell me how the trip went!" I said. "Was everyone just bowled over by the new you?"

She sighed, blinked back tears and said, "Sue, no one said a word."

"What?" I exclaimed. "What do you mean 'no one said a word'?"

"I mean just that," she said, looking dejected and disappointed. "It was like I hadn't changed at all. There was no comment. Not from my family, and not from my friends."

Imagine how upsetting that was to her. If someone really wanted to hurt her, they succeeded.

I gave her a big hug and had a flash of insight. "Are your family and friends overweight?" I asked.

"Yes, they are. Some of them are heavier than others but they could all stand to lose weight."

"Well there's your answer then. Your success just highlighted their problems," I explained. "They were embarrassed by their own weight problems and couldn't acknowledge your success because of it. I know you're upset and disappointed, but you can't let their problems become your problems. We all have enough of our own without taking on someone else's."

She laughed at that and said, "I know. It's okay. I'll be fine," and she was. She didn't let the episode derail her efforts but I'm sure the hurt travels with her over time.

Sabotage episodes like that are not easily forgotten. My own experience with the "silent treatment method of sabotage" will always be a sore spot in my heart.

After losing the weight, I registered with a research group called The National Weight Control Registry. These researchers from Pittsburgh compiled nutritional and exercise information on people who had lost at least thirty pounds and had kept the weight off for at least a year. They followed these successful "losers" over time to discover their strategies for weight loss and maintenance. (You too can be a part of the study if you have lost thirty pounds and kept it off for a year. See the footnote at the end of the book for further information.)

Sabotage: Don't Let Them See You Sweat

Agreeing to be in the study also means you may be approached for interviews by magazine and newspaper writers and publications penning weight loss pieces. By happenstance, Woman's Day magazine contacted me and I found myself and my weight loss story in a national publication. There was a before and after picture of myself, and information on how I had lost the weight.

I was thrilled. I was a celebrity! I went around and bought up a dozen copies of the Woman's Day issue from local outlets and sent them off to select family and friends. One person I sent it to was my father-in-law. Both of my parents, who had always been supportive of me, as well as my mother-in-law, were long dead and "Dad" was the only one left to enjoy my success. At least I assumed he would enjoy my success.

I mailed off the issue and waited for a response. I waited, and I waited, and there was no response. Finally, my husband called him and I asked him to ask if he had received the magazine. His response to my husband was, "Yes." Just "yes," nothing more. There was no "hip-hip-hurray"! There was no "congratulations." There was no "I'm so proud of you." There was nothing. No comment. Nothing. Nada. I was crushed, and I remain crushed to this day. Silence can cut as deeply as words sometimes.

I do not understand why someone would or could deprive another person of the obvious support and encouragement they need and deserve. It is, to me, a particularly mean thing to do. I naturally understood how the lady felt who got no response from her Christmastime reunion. But again, you need to realize that people do these things because of their own problems and not because of you. You cannot allow their insecurities and irrational responses to influence your weight loss efforts.

Find a diet coach or weight loss group, either online or not, for any support and encouragement you might need. Like-minded people will understand your pain in sabotage situations such as these, and they will give you the love and encouragement you need.

Weird as it seems, most times silence is the greatest compliment you can receive. When your best efforts, at anything, are met with silence, you can bet your accomplishment has been noticed.

Family Members As Saboteurs

It's obvious that friends can hurt us deeply, but family has even more power to sabotage our efforts. Obviously my father-in-law's silent treatment was damaging, but other relatives can be equally unsupportive. One young lady who had lost 12 pounds and didn't need to lose much more than that said she had worn a bikini the previous weekend for the first time in ages.

"My sister-in-law, who's a size 2, looked at me and said, 'Oh my. You have a lot of stretch marks showing.'"

"AHHHHHH," I said. "What did you say?"

"I've had five kids, Sue, so I told her, 'I guess the whole world will know I have children then.' She doesn't have any kids so I knew that would get her!"

Saboteurs better watch out whom they rile up.

I also have a story to relate. Before I lost my weight a certain family member was the thinnest person in the family. It took just one look at the new, improved me for her to hate me. Not that she didn't hate me before that, but she wasn't vicious when I was heavy. I didn't threaten her then.

We went to a family reunion together and my husband and I were into running at the time, and we could run many miles effortlessly. I asked if anyone wanted to run with us. This person's husband said, "No, she walks the hills at home but doesn't run."

Now I admit I responded most cattily, "People that can't run, walk." Boy, did that come back to haunt me.

Years later we visited these people for the first (and last) time and the "hills" which my family member walked were mountain slopes. The morning after our arrival I asked if she wanted to go for a walk. Their driveway and road from the highway was steep and I thought it would be a good incline to walk. She said, "Sure," and then advised me to take off my walking shoes. She then began to outfit me with socks and ill-fitting hiking boots. Naïve me should have realized I was in trouble.

We began to walk down her driveway but instead of continuing down the road we veered into the woods. I found myself on a steep incline of 30 degrees straight down, ankle deep in mud. The family member was making her way down the slippery incline sideways, planting her lower foot firmly in the mud while hollering at me, "One, and two! One, two. Come on! Step in time! One, two!" I thought she had morphed into a Nazi commando.

Rather than turn around and continue my walk in a civilized manner, I decided if she could do it, so could I. And I did. I trudged everywhere she went, which included getting us lost in the woods in waist high grass, complete with ticks, snakes, and God knows what else. I matched her step for step, through shoe-sucking mud and small rivers, crawling under brambles, and trudging through "trails" that disappeared at regular intervals.

I avoided as much poison ivy as possible. Being highly allergic to it, that was my worst fear. I'm not sure she even knew what it looked like or she would have made sure I walked right through it. I did know she certainly didn't know where we were. Getting lost in the wilderness with Miss Gestapo was my second worst fear.

Eventually, several hours later and after doing several switchbacks, she managed to find our way back to her house, but only with the help of her dogs, which located us and showed us the way home. The final test was to climb up a nearly vertical incline into their backyard, which I also managed to accomplish even with the ill-fitting shoes. Upon seeing my husband he asked, "How was your walk?"

As I wiped dripping sweat from the end of my nose, blotted the blood running down my legs, and picked burrs out of my hair I said, "Your stinking relative tried to kill me."

He thought I was kidding and to this day only she and I really know what went on in those woods but believe me when I tell you it was the nastiest, most mean-spirited thing anyone has ever done to me, and that is saying a lot. I have never done anything to her to deserve such treatment. Except make one catty remark; oh, and lose a lot of weight!

Since this woman is deathly afraid of the water, I anxiously await her arrival to our tropical home where I intend to take her out to the reef several miles offshore and leave her there. Perhaps I'll leave her some nice bloody chum so she can feed my friends, the sharks and barracudas.

What do you think was her motivation for that "excursion" through the woods? What purpose did it serve, in her mind? I can only figure she was jealous and wanted to put me in my place. She's a perfect example of people resenting your success and happiness.

Don't be surprised to find that your success threatens other people. And I'm not just talking about losing weight, here. When you are successful in any way, certain people will strive to change that. Sometimes, though, it is an innocent comment that does the most damage because it is hard to detect it as sabotage. A passing, yet cutting, remark from someone close to us can easily derail our weight loss efforts.

For example, Karen told me, "I once weighed 138. Just once. But when I did, my mother said to me, 'You look so old since you lost all that weight.' The next time I stepped on the scale I weighed 162 and I thought to myself, 'I guess I don't look so old anymore.'"

Mothers are apparently frequent saboteurs. My mother didn't do this to me, so I understand this to be true from the people I have counseled. A successful lawyer recounts how her mother used to clip out articles from magazines and newspapers about the health dangers of obesity and give them to her. (And she's not even close to being obese.) Imagine the warped body image this behavior created in her daughter.

Food Pushers

There are also stories of mothers preparing favorite dishes for their dieting children and then saying, "But you have to eat some. It's your favorite. I made it just for you". This behavior is called "food pushing" and I am guilty of it myself so I'm going to defend it.

Being a mother, and a "foodie" myself, I understand this nurturing tendency. I, too, love to feed people. However, food pushing is definitely a form of sabotage.

This type of sabotage I can almost forgive. It's like a test. Tempting us allows us to show our resolve and let our family know the importance of our newfound healthy eating habits. Nevertheless, we need to understand that many of our cultures and family environments use food as a means to show love for special people.

The Christmas cookies that Grandma made just for you and the macaroni and cheese that made you feel so much better as a child when you were sick are all magic potients that spell L-O-V-E. It's easy to understand why we grew up overweight when we take a nutrient and imbue it with emotional capabilities. Food is merely for sustenance. Relationships and love are for emotional well-being. Still, food is a special substance and its preparation does require love.

Turning down a portion of L-O-V-E would be unthinkable, and turning down a portion of Mom's apple pie may be, too. People may think it rude to not eat something made especially for you, and others may think it's a form of rejection. If you cannot feign being full and ask to take the food home with you (to later be fed to the dog or given to your roommate), then take the advice of Emily Post who said, "The correct response to a food pusher is, 'No.' The polite response is 'No, thank you.'"

Maria is a dieter who fully recognizes herself as a compulsive overeater. Unfortunately, she has a sister who is a food pusher. The combination of family member and food pusher is deadly. Maria is always blaming her sister for her own lack of control and overeating. The sister always comes to visit with an array of tempting pies. They are her specialty and Maria cannot, and will not, resist eating them. So who's at fault here? Obviously both of them are guilty and both of them (excuse the pun) feed off of one another's faults.

Remember that the most hurtful thing about sabotage is that we are blindsided by it. It is not expected. It comes from unlikely sources at unlikely times, but it is always because our new habits, lifestyle, or appearance is threatening to someone. Nasty, vindictive people are everywhere. Don't let them interfere with your efforts to reach your goals. I like to say "the best revenge is living well," and it's true. You can get your revenge calmly and easily by losing the weight, getting fit and trim, being active and healthy and beautiful, and above all by enjoying yourself. It gets them every time.

The Ultimate Saboteur: The Spouse (Or Significant Other)

Spousal sabotage is the very worst kind. The people we live with present special problems. Husbands and wives sometimes become saboteurs when they see their spouses losing weight and changing before their very eyes. A supportive husband that sees his wife become attractive to other men can sometimes become a saboteur overnight. Likewise a supportive wife may have second thoughts when she sees her newly trim husband interact with other women.

Many "significant others" try to avoid the whole scenario by telling their loved ones that they "like you heavy because there's more to love." This response is an effort to keep the status quo. A pleasingly plump spouse may be a spouse that stays close to home. This refrain also is a form of sabotage in itself because it can keep a person from pursuing the goal they set for themselves.

Sabotage that comes from spouses is particularly damaging. One longtime friend comes to mind when I think about unsupportive husbands. This lovely lady was really on a roll, steadily losing weight and walking her way to a healthy and fit body. Then, the struggle became too much for her and I wondered what had happened. The truth came out when she said, "My husband isn't supporting me."

"What is he doing?"

"Well, believe it or not, he actually left a note on the kitchen counter for me that said, 'You are spending too much time and effort trying to lose this weight. I want all this counting calories and dieting and you walking every day to stop, and stop now.'"

"He left a note? A written note? What did you do?"

"I left him a note that said, 'Eat s--t and die.'"

Everyone within earshot became hushed and silent as most of our mouths dropped to the floor, then, the lady next to me leans over to me and asks, "How many calories is that?"

I burst out laughing and to this day find that episode remains one of the funniest things I've ever heard.

Of course, the true problem wasn't funny at all. That a husband, a trusted companion and loved one, would go to such lengths to sabotage someone's sincere effort to better themselves is unconscionable. The sheer hurtfulness is hard for me to comprehend, much less understand.

The sad truth is that he accomplished what he set out to do. My friend gained back the weight she had lost and continues to struggle with her desire to lose the weight and her husband's opposition to her efforts.

There's also a most wonderful man who comes to mind when I think about unsupportive spouses. This guy is the sweetest, kindest, most hard-working man you'll ever meet. He has successfully lost weight before but mostly through a quick-fix type of attitude, which is very typical for a man. He has never reached the point where healthy eating is truly a lifestyle change. But he does keep trying.

The biggest obstacle to his success is his wife and daughter who constantly berate him about his appearance, even when he's successfully taking the weight off. The final straw that usually ends his weight loss efforts is when his family begins to police his food consumption. This is a competent man, not a child who needs policing. Their attitude undermines his feeling that he is in control of his eating and it spells the end of his attempts.

Spouses oftentimes act this way. They become "the food police." I don't know why they do it, but they do. They know you are watching your food intake and something suddenly requires them to ask, "Are you sure you can eat that?" or "That's not on your diet. You can't have that!"

Naturally, telling us what we can and cannot do is the surest way to make us rebel. No one wants to be policed and it is unnecessary because you can eat whatever you want when you are trying to lose weight, so long as you compensate for it somewhere else. Try to be patient with them and with yourself. Ignore them or educate them. It's your choice. Just don't let them sabotage you.

Usually, recognizing the motivation behind spousal sabotage can lead to a better understanding between couples. If a spouse fears a change in environment (i.e. she'll never be able to eat chicken wings again because her husband's on a diet), or fears losing your love and attention, then these are issues that can be addressed. Sometimes involving a spouse fully in the weight loss effort can lead to better support. You are both going to eat healthier and lower your cholesterol readings, for instance, or you are both going to take ballroom dance lessons for some fun and exercise.

On the other hand, sometimes keeping your weight loss efforts a secret from your spouse is a better tactic. If you are the one buying and preparing the food it's quite possible that you can change the menu and meal preparation to healthier options without your spouse even knowing about it. Letting your significant other know your weight loss intentions or not really depends on the spouse. Usually, though, open and honest discussion leads to negotiating a more supportive environment.

Negotiating a supportive environment and eliminating any sabotage first requires that you define the problem and the person causing it. Then you have to think about what kind of support you need from that person. Maybe you need your husband to take the children for a few hours each Saturday morning while you go to the gym. That's a specific request that he can satisfy. Asking him to "be more supportive" is too nebulous. You must be specific and direct. This applies to asking men for what you want in all areas, not just weight loss. Be direct. Be specific. Be concise. You will get what you want more often than not.

If your skinny husband asks you to get him a bowl of ice cream every night after dinner and you are dipping a spoon into the ice cream container and eating some yourself while you dip his, then you have a problem. Tell him directly that you cannot resist that temptation and he has to get his ice cream himself for the next three months. Again, be specific! Don't let him think he has to do it forever; just three months is all you ask of him. He'll oblige.

You could ask your mother not to make the Double Dutch Chocolate Cake (which you cannot resist) but instead make her world famous Chicken Cacciatore (which you can figure the calorie count for). Be specific! You don't necessarily have to be terribly truthful, either. Tell Mom the chocolate may trigger a headache or you have to get up early the next day and it keeps you awake. Sometimes linking the request to something other than your diet is much more readily accepted because people then don't think you are imposing your dietary restrictions on them.

Self-Sabotage

There are also many times when we sabotage ourselves. Red light foods make their way into our grocery carts and then enter our houses; we drink a little too much at a special dinner out and find our best intentions to eat healthy fade away with our inhibitions; and sometimes we simply lose our focus and give in to temptation.

"I felt like a rebellious teenager," said one young woman who had just recently reached her weight goal and found it difficult to stay motivated. "I simply didn't care what I ate and I gained four pounds in no time flat."

In the diet war you have to be your own ally, not your own worst enemy. If you are not taking steps to lose weight and be healthier for yourself and no one else, then the effort becomes a monumental struggle and you will sabotage yourself. You will sabotage yourself because the struggle requires too much effort and too much time. When you do it all for yourself; for your own appearance, and your own fitness, and your own self-esteem, and your own sense of well-being, then it becomes less of a struggle and more of a crusade. It suddenly takes less effort and becomes easier to stay in control.

Finally, be grateful for all the support you do receive. By and large, most people will help you in your endeavor and be happy for you and proud of your accomplishments. Anyone who resents your success has problems which you should not take on as your own.

If all else fails and your support system falls apart, please find a support group or a diet coach. Both provide compassion, support, and advice. You can also visit the "Win When You Lose" Facebook page to interact with people who share your concerns and problems. Speak up and let everyone know what you are going through and allow them to help you sort it out. That's what they are there for. Chances are you'll find another person that has gone through the exact same experience and has the solution to your problem.

Things to remember from this chapter:

- Your success triggers all kinds of insecurities in other people. Many times those insecurities are manifested as sabotage.

- Sabotage comes from people you trust, when you least expect it, which makes it particularly hurtful and damaging.

- Find a diet coach, group support system, our Facebook group, or like-minded friends to provide you with encouragement and understanding, as well as advice in challenging situations.

- Food pushing is a common form of sabotage.

- Food policing is a common form of sabotage.

- Spousal sabotage is the worst kind, but you can usually negotiate a supportive environment with a spouse/significant other.

- Living well is the best revenge.

Chapter 5 – Self-Esteem

So how does low self-esteem due to weight issues affect your life? To answer this question, first think about what we would have done or tried to do in our lives if weight had not been an obstacle. What activities would we have tried? What people would we have met or approached? What confrontations would we have initiated? What emotions would we have expressed? What professional opportunities would we have we pursued?

I posed this question and the responses were enlightening.

"I would have tried sky-diving," said one person.

"I would have worn a bikini!" several ladies blurted out simultaneously.

"I would have kicked my lousy husband to the curb long before I actually did!" came a voice from the back of the room.

Everyone laughed, but we appreciated the sentiment behind the response. The lady in question meant that she would have had the self-confidence and strength to change an uncomfortable situation if she had been happier within herself.

Being overweight often demeans us in our own eyes. Unfortunately, it also demeans us in the eyes of employers, family, and friends. It keeps us from enjoying life in a host of different ways.

Hesitance To try New Activities

Weight issues hold us back from trying new and unusual physical activities. Being overweight makes us feel ungainly and less than agile. Just the other week I suggested waterskiing as a fun activity and someone said something about not being able to "haul my bulk out of the water." I fully understood the trepidation, but encouraged them to attempt it and see for themselves rather than make an assumption that would prevent them from trying something new. Think about all the opportunities you've missed because you felt ashamed and embarrassed by your weight. Don't let another opportunity pass you by.

One notable lady lives in Florida with easy access to the beach as well as a backyard pool. Yet she refuses to take advantage of these offerings, saying, "I can't let anyone see me in a swimsuit." While I understand her emotion, I do think it is a form of masochism to deny yourself the simple pleasures of life because you are ashamed of your body.

You can go to the beach and never see a soul you know, so who cares how your swimsuit fits? Lots of other people on the beach have less than perfect bodies. And in your own backyard you should be comfortable in your own element. The upside rationalization is that the exercise you get walking the beach or splashing in the pool will ultimately make you look better in the swimsuit you despise so much.

When I mentioned kayaking I heard, "Can't you get stuck in those things? I'm sure I'd get stuck in one." The gentleman assumed a modern kayak requires you to be inside it when you really sit on top of most of them. You will not get stuck in a kayak. Try it; you'll love it.

Our reluctance to participate in athletic activities can sometimes be traced back to early childhood experiences. If you were overweight in grade school, you were surely ridiculed.

Gym Class

When I was in elementary school I had a terrible time fitting in with the other children because of my weight. I was ridiculed and teased unmercifully, but the worst abuse I endured was at the hands of the gym teacher.

An older man with glasses and snow-white hair, he appeared kindly at first glance. I doubt anyone other than the kids in his gym class really knew what a sadist he truly was. My feeling now is that he concealed his true self quite well among the staff and administrators. Of course at the time, I was a mere first, second, third, etc. grader who was entirely powerless against this individual. In those days, you had the same gym teacher for your entire stay in elementary school so I put up with this man for five long years. Thankfully, he left in my sixth year.

At the time, President John F. Kennedy enacted the "President's Council on Physical Fitness." This program required children to perform a battery of physical fitness tasks, scores were recorded, and the school (I presume) was judged according to how many kids performed at or above the prescribed fitness levels.

Among the fitness feats were chin-ups, sit-ups, the monkey bars, sit and reach, and various running distances including the 600 yard dash. Needless to say, I performed most of those feats miserably. Some of them I could do pretty well. I was good at sit-ups and I was flexible enough to exceed the sit and reach standards. That, however, was not enough to prevent this man from calling me "jelly- belly," "fat-so," "lard ass" and any other derogatory remark he could think of.

I vividly recall two incidents, one of which I'll share with you here. Everyone set out to valiantly complete that 600 yard dash. We all took off around the perimeter of the playing fields while Mr. Sadist stood in the center of the baseball diamond and perused our progress.

Towards the end I had an unbearably painful stitch in my side and pain in my right knee, but I knew I couldn't quit. My only intent was to finish well enough to avoid ridicule from this man.

Unfortunately, I couldn't. Other kids had finished the run and were laying at the finish line trying to catch their breath as I turned the corner and saw them there. Suddenly, Mr. Sadist was running towards me, and then he was running beside me as I gasped and stumbled.

"Come on Jelly-Belly! You can't finish. I know you can't. You're too fat to even run! HAHAHA. Here comes Jelly-Belly kids. Thank her for ruining your scores. May as well just write "didn't finish" here instead of recording a time. Yours is so slow it doesn't even count."

I was totally humiliated. To this day, forty-odd years later, I can hear his words exactly and see the laughing, taunting faces of the students against the backdrop of a cloudless blue sky and a vividly green ball field. I can feel the pain in my side and in my knee and I can feel the sting of tears.

Today this man would, hopefully, be jailed for child abuse. But he shaped my feelings about myself. I believed for most of my life that I was uncoordinated and ungainly. I was totally unathletic and would be an embarrassment to my team, my coach, and myself if I tried any athletic endeavor. Plus, I was fat.

I shared this story to a group of people and expected others to commiserate with me and tell everyone about experiences they had had as children. I was surprised to be met with mostly silence. Maybe those childhood traumas are just too painful for most people to revisit. Two people did go back, though.

Gary talked about how the worst thing for him was trying to climb to the top of the rope in junior high school. "Everyone would stand around and watch you and jeer at you. Most of the guys shinnied up that rope without any problem but if you were heavy, it was harder to use your upper body to pull your lower body up." Gary had a smile on his face as he told the story, but you could see the hurt of that experience underneath the grin.

"Then things changed when you got to high school! Suddenly they wanted you to be heavy so you could be on the football team!" he exclaimed, shaking his head incredulously.

"That's the way it was for boys," Cherie said. "It just got harder for girls in high school. We were expected to be even thinner. There's never been a time when being a heavy girl has been acceptable, encouraged, or even tolerated."

At another venue I got a soulful look and a nodding head from a lady as I told my story. "Can you relate to this?" I asked her after I had finished.

"Oh yes. It was always like that for me in school. I never fit in because of my weight."

I tried to get her to elaborate but she wouldn't open up any more than that. It was obviously too painful to recall.

Childhood experiences color our perceptions of ourselves and affect our self-esteem in far-reaching ways. Painful childhood memories of gym class are often what hold us back from being athletic adults.

Expressing Yourself

We need to remember we are no longer that powerless child that was so harshly criticized. At the time we had to hold our tongues or risk being sent to the principal's office, but now we are grown adults. We can look back and realize that our gym teacher was, guess what?, Fat! I would relish seeing him on the street today so I could tell him just what I think of him. I can even do that without actually seeing him. I can do that in my mind, where most powerful thoughts and emotions take shape. Expressing yourself either mentally or verbally empowers you.

What other ways of expressing yourself would you choose if you were sure of yourself and less self-conscious?

"I've been in love with a certain person for years, but I have never felt worthy of them because of my weight. I'm sure they wouldn't look twice at me the way I am," said one twenty-something young woman. She weighed about 300 pounds at the time.

It's easy to understand her misgivings about expressing her feelings to this man. She is unsure of herself, afraid of being rejected, and so she does nothing. But even if she loses the weight she will still be afraid of being rejected. The only difference may be her self-esteem raises enough to allow her to approach him at all.

Sara chimed in. "My problem was just the opposite. I had the man and needed to get rid of him! He was toxic to me and I knew it, but I was afraid of being alone and thought no one else would ever want to be with me."

"You said 'had' the man," I noted. "What happened?"

"Oh, I eventually lost the weight, regained my self-worth, and divorced him. Then, just like everyone always says, when I wasn't looking, I stumbled onto the love of my life. We've been together for 15 years."

Losing weight is so empowering. Stories of people taking control of their lives after taking control of their diets never cease to inspire me.

"I used to be rather timid," said one boisterous lady.

"You? Timid?"

"Oh yeah," she replied. "I never confronted anyone, never really expressed myself. I was too afraid no one would love me if I exposed my true feelings. But once I lost the weight and felt better in my own skin, I became who I am today."

I smiled, thinking how she told me a thing or two once or twice when I was wrong about something. She was definitely no longer a timid character. Good for her. We should all be comfortable expressing ourselves, regardless of our weight. Yet being at your ideal weight allows you to find your own voice in many different instances.

Professional Limitations

Perhaps the most poignant response to my initial question, 'How has being overweight limited your life?' came from a gentleman who said, "I would have been more successful at my work."

I couldn't let that comment pass by without a discussion so I asked, "In what way would you have been more successful?"

"Well I used to be an executive for a Fortune 500 company. We were told that 'Thin is in and stout is out,' meaning that anyone overweight did not project the kind of image that the corporation was looking for. Only thin and trim men were chosen to make presentations to clients, for example. I know for sure that I was passed over for advancement and promotions because of my weight."

I silently wondered if he could have pleaded his case with his employer if he had been more self-confident. Otherwise, a discrimination lawsuit seemed obvious, but only an empowered individual could mount that kind of confrontation.

Then Emily told a story about her son. "He's over 400 pounds but he's losing weight steadily right now. A while back he applied for a job as a computer programmer and he told me he knew instantly that he would not get the job when he arrived

75

for the interview. He said the surprised look on the interviewer's face was a dead giveaway. And he has a Master's Degree in Computer Science and would have been perfect for that job. His education and experience couldn't overcome his appearance." You could feel a mother's pain for her son's ordeal as she told this story.

The social consequences of being overweight are not ignored by people with weight problems, but they are seldom discussed openly simply because the experiences are so painful.

Family And Friends

My father had a friend, an old crusty farmer type who chewed tobacco and wore mud caked work boots no matter where he was or what the circumstance. This man used to call me a "little heifer" as in, "Well she's a cute little heifer."

My father never said a word in my defense. Again, I internalized that comment and thought of myself as a fat cow for many years afterwards. Twenty-five years passed before I saw that man again. I was in the company of my oldest brother, Paul. Paul spoke to the man and said to him, "You know Susie, Al." And to me, "Susie, this is Al Tarturrom."

I extended my hand and said, "Oh sure, I know Al," as I stood there at 127 pounds in a clingy tank top and short shorts.

When Al could finally pull his tongue back into his mouth and pick his jaw up off of the floor he responded with, "THIS is Susie?"

That was a very satisfying moment. Seeing that old coot much older, fatter, and dumbstruck was ample reward for losing the weight and finally realizing that my heifer days were over.

Complete Strangers

Derision doesn't always come from people you know well, of course. It seems to hurt more when it comes from someone with whom you share some history, though. Nevertheless, complete strangers can wield their own power over us if we give them that opportunity.

"I went into a department store and I was looking at size 14 dresses when a salesperson approached me and said, 'You don't belong in here. You need to go over to the Plus-size department in the back there.'", related Martha. "Now how did she know I wasn't looking to buy something for someone else, or for a thinner "me" for that matter? I was so hurt and humiliated that I didn't even say a word to her. I just got out of there in a hurry."

Notice that Martha "didn't say a word to her." Again, we are afraid to express ourselves when our self-esteem is low.

I had a similar experience while shopping. A salesperson came up to me while I was browsing for something for someone else and said," You're not thinking there's anything in this department to fit you, are you?" I was so stunned I can't even remember what I said back to her, but I recall the painful feeling vividly. I also know I said something back to her. Anything.

Similarly, complete strangers often comment on our food choices. I have no idea why they do this.

One night my husband and I went to dinner at a local casual dining establishment. We had to wait for a table and rather than wait at the bar, drinking, we chose to sit outside and catch up on the day's events.

I could see through the window into the dining room and noticed one table of six people. They ordered several appealing (read: fattening) appetizers, tropical drinks, entrees, and then desserts. I noticed because I had skimped on food all day long to be able to eat dinner at this place and I wanted a table as soon as possible.

When we were finally seated I ordered first. I ordered a cup of conch chowder (tomato-based and similar to clam chowder), a garden salad with honey-mustard dressing on the side, and a hamburger. The waitress got a funny look on her face as I recited my choices to her. She stopped writing, looked down at her feet, and finally said, "You know, that's a lot of food."

I was shocked! I wanted to scream out, "Why aren't you telling that to that table over there?????"

I assume she meant well in telling me that but this was my dinner and my choices. I was taking steps to make it healthy and I did not need or ask for her commentary on my food choices. This critiquing happens quite often to me. I don't like it and I express myself with a paltry tip if I leave one at all.

Self-Esteem Contrasted With Self-Image

It's these judgments by society that cause us to associate self-esteem and self-image with body- image and weight. Breaking this association is one of the keys to successful weight loss and management. Sharing our experiences and voicing our pain illuminates the idiocy of such situations. It reveals that we have all experienced societal disdain and we should not accept it in the future.

Certain roles models of larger sizes are becoming more apparent in the media. Oprah, Queen Latifah, Emme (a plus size model) and Carre Otis (a once rail thin model who is now a more healthy and realistic weight) can all help society overcome these obstacles, but what about us as individuals? Do we plan to perpetuate and contribute to the discrimination by allowing it to hamper our growth and life experiences? Would we chastise and discriminate against others because of their weight? If not, then we should certainly not do it to ourselves.

I feel I must mention here that I have a very slender husband (more about him later!) who also feels discriminated against because of his body shape and style. While those of us who struggle with our weight may feel unjustly judged, be aware that thin people are as much out of place in our society as heavy ones, perhaps more so as the whole of society becomes more overweight.

Don't let yourself become the type of judgmental person we have struggled against our whole lives. Reverse discrimination is discrimination nonetheless. We can certainly be jealous of our naturally thin friends and family but their body composition may be as much as a problem for them as ours is to us. Be compassionate.

Right now there is a woman named Bethenny Frankel who is promoting herself and various products as "Skinny Girl." Personally, I enjoy Bethenny and applaud her success. I think her empowering message to all women is inspiring and her ambition is admirable.

However, I do not think she has ever had a weight problem. In fact, I think she is obsessed with being thin. My point is that people I know with weight problems have voiced unwarranted criticism of her because she is so thin, seemingly effortlessly. That criticism stems from jealousy. There should be no room for that kind of thinking in our heads. It is detrimental and we, who have been judged our whole lives by our weight, should know better than to do that to someone else. Go Bethenny! You have my utmost respect for your accomplishments.

The Vicious Cycle

Being overweight lowers our self-esteem and our lowered self-esteem perpetuates our being overweight. Breaking the connection is what we need to do.

You Can Do, You Can Do

You must feel that you deserve to be fit and trim and healthy in order to become that way. Knowing that you can accomplish the transformation is the second step. By comparison, actually doing it is the easy part.

I wish I could show you the transformations that I have seen firsthand when people lose the weight. I have witnessed unbelievable evolutions as people rediscover themselves and what they can accomplish. Timidity gives way to outspokenness; many times baggy clothes change into shape-hugging, brightly colored creations; hairstyles change and sometimes hair color, too; frowns are replaced with smiles; a sluggish gait becomes a lively step; shy personalities transform into gregariousness; and beautiful butterflies emerge from the cocoon of weight.

You deserve to be happy and you deserve to reach your goals. It's as simple as that. Furthermore, you are perfect right now at whatever weight you carry. The problem is that you don't know that to be true. But you will as soon as you give yourself the opportunity to regain control of your life, your health, your weight, your eating, and your self-image.

Things to remember from this chapter:

- Being overweight lowers our self-esteem and lowered self-esteem perpetuates our being overweight. Break the connection!

- Low self-esteem restricts us from trying new activities, expressing ourselves, being successful, reaching for new heights.

- Everyone has painful childhood memories but they do not let them define them. You are no longer a defenseless child. You are now a capable adult.

- Everyone; family, friends, and perfect strangers can undermine your self-esteem if you allow them to do so. In many cases, your success triggers all kinds of insecurities in other people, which they then foist on you.

- When you find your ideal weight you will also find your own voice.

- You deserve to be fit and trim and healthy.

Chapter 6 - Exercise

Another way to add to your burgeoning self-esteem is to incorporate exercise into your everyday routine. There was a time not so long ago when we did not use the "E" word. Instead, we used the "A" word: Activity. The ban on the word "exercise" still exists to some extent and for good reason. As soon as "exercise" becomes the topic of conversation, people tend to get nervous.

Activity, however, connotes less of a structured effort and more of a gentle approach to movement. Exercise per se sometimes conjures memories of our school gym classes where we were taunted and shunned. How many of us were the last ones chosen for kickball or dodge ball or basketball? I rest my case. (See the subsection of the Self-Esteem chapter for more about these issues.)

Make It Play

Similar to the differences between exercise and activity is the difference between activity and play. Play connotes even more of a fun-filled experience than activity does. Think about when you were in grade school. You came bounding in the door after school, relieved to be home and excited to have a few hours of unstructured time, grabbed a doughnut probably, and said, "Hi Mom, I'm home. I'm going out to exercise now." Is that what you said? Your attitude about exercise is a powerful thing. It can either encourage you or deter you.

If we could just recapture that playful attitude we enjoyed as kids towards the simple movement of our bodies, our weight loss and management would be much easier. If you really think about what activities you enjoyed as children, you may find a clue to what you'd enjoy as adults. Did you like to ride your bike? Did you enjoy playing on a softball team? How much fun was skipping rope or roller- skating? Maybe you loved to swim.

One of the most important things you can do for your health, your weight, your self-esteem, and your attitude is to find some sort of physical activity that you enjoy. If you hate the regiment required to go to the gym and find yourself surrounded by people that belong in a Met-X commercial, just don't do it. How disheartening to make yourself do something you despise.

Walking

Walking seems to be the preferred method of adding activity to your day right now. It's easy, doesn't require expensive equipment (except for a good pair of sturdy shoes), and you can do it anywhere and anytime. It's also totally adaptable to your fitness level. You can stroll a few blocks when you start out and work your way up to walking at a faster pace, or maybe even jogging, for longer distances. In this way there is visible and measurable evidence of your progress that serves to motivate you to higher achievements.

Tracking your walking progress is a great motivator, too. Just jot down on your calendar or note on your phone how long and how far you walk each day. Try to gently increase the time, distance, or intensity over the course of a month. You'll be surprised to see how far you have come after 30 days.

You have probably heard that we should all get 10,000 steps a day into our regular routine. This milestone is an admirable one, and one we should all strive to achieve. A pedometer goes a long way to encouraging the 10,000 step ideal. Walking across the parking lot, walking up the stairs, walking around when you are on the phone, all help you reach that goal. However, don't stress out about it. It's great to have that goal, but it might be too much to reach for if you are starting out at zero. Just start slowly and work up to it.

Walking has other side benefits, too. It gets you out of the house and away from the television. It's a fabulous stress reliever that allows you to clear your head even when emotions run high. It's an activity you can do with others. Walking groups are popular, but you also might get your spouse to join you and your dogs would certainly appreciate the outing. Similarly, walking with your children can make it family time and a way and catch up on what happened in everyone's day.

Walking is a great all-round way to get into shape and it's fun, too. You might want to listen to some music or maybe even a book on tape as you set out. The music can set the pace of your walk and soothe your frazzled nerves and a book may be a way for you to make the time truly your own.

Just getting out into the world has its own rewards. The change of season will become more evident to you as you notice how the trees are changing and the air feels. You'll meet your neighbors, both human and otherwise. I always carry a pocket full of dog treats so I know all the neighborhood canine residents. Visiting with them as I go on my way makes it more enjoyable.

Other Activity

Walking is only one suggestion for an enjoyable activity. Plenty of other choices exist. Younger people in my meetings gravitate towards rollerblading. In our climate, water aerobics, swimming, snorkeling, diving, and other related water sports all help keep our weight under control. Paddle-boarding is the newest craze. You stand on what is essentially a surfboard in calm water and paddle yourself around. It is wonderful exercise for your "core" muscles like your abdominals, as well as your arms. Tennis and golf also entice many people to get out and "play."

One of my favorite things to do is to take my dog to agility class. She jumps through hoops, and goes over jumps, and dashes through tunnels; meanwhile, I sweat, and jog beside her, and generally get an amazing workout myself. I am huffing and puffing in no time, but the "play" element makes it all bearable.

It really doesn't matter what activity you choose. The most important thing is to simply choose one, and make it one that you enjoy. The second most important thing to remember is consistency is all-important. What you do doesn't matter so much as the fact that you do it on a regular basis. Two days a week of exercise will not keep your weight in check. You need to do your chosen activity five or six days a week, consistently.

That said, there are many, many books extolling the benefits of regular exercise. They all are valuable resources to motivate you and guide you. The exercise routines they contain may help you progress from one fitness level to another in a safe manner. You don't want to overdo and hurt yourself the first few times out. That won't help you be consistent or progress. Taking the advice of exercise professionals is a very good idea. Even investing in time with a personal trainer (with good credentials) may be the key to your weight loss and exercise success. You should also ask for your doctor's advice and consent before starting any physical activity plan.

Determining Calorie Expenditure

There's a structured way to determine how effectively you are burning calories. It requires you to identify three pieces of information. You first have to determine the intensity of the activity, then the duration, and finally your own body weight.

Determining the intensity of the activity is easy. The medical and exercise communities have devised this simple evaluation tool: if you can still sing while you are doing the activity and you will not break a sweat then you are exercising at a light intensity; if you can talk but not sing and you break a sweat after ten minutes of continuous activity then you are said to be working at a moderate level of intensity; and lastly, if you can speak only briefly but not carry on a conversation at all and you are sweating after several minutes of activity you are said to be working at a high intensity.

These intensity levels, combined with duration of the activity and your body weight indicate how many calories you are burning in a given exercise period. This formula is why you burn more calories at a heavier weight than you do after losing 20 pounds, for example. As you lose weight, you have to adjust your exercise goals accordingly, or cut back on your food intake. It's all very scientific and rational. There are many formulas available that use this information to determine what you can eat in return for what you have earned through exercise.

Don't Move More To Eat; Move More To Be Happier

My advice is different. Just get out and move most every day of the week for the sheer pleasure and stress-management benefits of activity. Do not think you can eat more because you have moved more. Try very hard to make movement part of who you are and you will be a huge step closer to being healthier and leaner.

One time a stylish young woman tentatively approached me. She and I had not had much interaction before this conversation.

"Ahhhh, Sue, can I ask you a question?" she asked as she looked around nervously.

"Sure Sandy. How are you?" I responded.

"I'm OK," she said, "I just have a question about this activity stuff."

I waited patiently for her to continue, wondering what question she might have for me when she blurted out, "Is sex considered an activity and how many calories do you think you use doing it?"

I thought about my own sex life and decided I had neglected to count a big expenditure of calories as activity. How clever Sandy was! I said, "Oh sure! And I'm glad you've found an enjoyable way to incorporate activity into your day."

She smiled, but I could tell she was still embarrassed by her question. Nevertheless she pressed the point, "How can you figure your calorie expenditure, then?"

I took a deep breath and decided the best way to approach this question would be just like I would approach any other exercise question. "Well you have to determine the intensity of the effort first.

OK, now what intensity would you say you're experiencing?" I asked innocently. It was all I could do not to laugh out loud.

"Oh it's definitely intense for five or ten minutes," she whispered.

Trying desperately to keep a straight face I said, "Then let's use that in our calculations."

"But what about the rest of the time?"

"You'll have to do a separate calculation for that time and evaluate your intensity level again," I responded.

"Well plug in 20 minutes of moderate intensity and another 20 minutes of light intensity," she said.

We finally figured out that her lovemaking session was using up about 150 calories.

"What?!?!" she exclaimed. "I think it should be a whole lot more than that."

"You go home and work on extending that high intensity level for at least twenty minutes then," I laughed.

"It's not me you have to talk to," she moaned. "It's my husband!" At which point we both burst into laughter with knowing glances and a twinkle in our eyes.

The moral of the story is exercise is exercise. Find what you enjoy and do it often. And don't worry about the calorie expenditure. Just believe that the movement is good for you and good for your weight loss efforts, too.

Things to remember from this chapter:

- Don't think of it as exercise, think of it as activity.

- Better yet, think of it as play!

- Find what you like to do and do it five days a week.

- Consistency is key.

- Exercise for the benefits it provides, not so that you can eat more.

Chapter 7 – Think Thin

There's a demonstration sometimes used in college classrooms to demonstrate time management. It is a great demonstration because of the visual impact and the lingering memory. People have told me years later that they often think of this demonstration under varying circumstances.

Time Management

First, a large vase is shown. The vase represents the viewer's life. To the vase I added about four inches of pebbles. I say, "These pebbles represent all the demands on your time made by work, family, chores, errands, etc." Then four ping pong balls are dropped into the vase. "These ping pong balls represent your needs. This one is for your health. This one is for your happiness through hobbies and interests. This one is for your emotional needs. Oops, that one doesn't quite fit. And there is one left over. This one represents your relationships, but it doesn't fit in at all. OK. Let's see if we can rearrange things a little."

Everything is then dumped out of the vase. This time I add a ping pong ball. "There's your health. Now let's put in your interests and happiness." In goes another ping pong ball. "Now let's add some responsibilities to others." Some pebbles are added which fall between the cracks and crevices created by the ping pong balls. "Now let's try to fit in some more of your needs," I say as I put in another ball. Then I'd drop in some more pebbles and finally the final ball. Everything fit quite nicely in the vessel.

My question was, "What's the moral of the story?"

The most memorable response to that question was, "The moral of the story is the big balls always go in first!"

91

Naturally, I completely lost my composure and everyone erupted into laughter. Still, the message was received that when you take care of yourself first you then have the resources you need to take care of all the other people and things in your life that demand your attention. Just like the pebbles and the ping pong balls, if your needs come first, then everything else falls into place.

A national weight loss center used to have a slogan: "When I control my weight I also control my life."

The slogan and the demonstration are the same. Taking care of yourself allows you to take care of everything else. Now what does that have to do with "Think Thin?" you ask. I believe it has everything to do with it.

Thin People Make "Me Time"

In my experience, I have observed that most thin people, and I refer to those that work at being thin, not those divinely blessed with thinness, adhere to this "me first" philosophy. You see them taking the time out of their schedules to walk or jog or bike ride or take a yoga class. They nourish themselves through hobbies and sports. They read. And they don't feel guilty about it, either! And really, why should they?

Sure we all have things we need to accomplish. We all have demands on our time and other people depending on us. But in the grand scheme of things, who is going to tend to those things and those needs if we are incapacitated? If we let our health and weight doom us to diabetes and cancer and heart disease, who then will pick up the slack our illness creates? Isn't it much better to take care of ourselves first and avoid those consequences?

I've always believed that most overweight people are born caretakers and people-pleasers. They nurture and baby and generally give of themselves to others long before they will give to themselves. Additionally, a great majority, though not all by any means, of overweight people are type -A personalities. They're the ones that get on the treadmill at home and find themselves looking around the room. What they see is dust, piles of papers that need sorting, bills that need paying, and a clock which says they really should be fixing dinner or doing the laundry rather than devoting time and energy to themselves.

Conversely, thin people give to themselves first and then turn their attention to others. It's a behavior we should try to emulate when we ourselves are attempting to lose weight. All the other little details and demands of life can wait. They will still be there after your exercise session. Using them as an excuse to deny yourself the time to be healthy and fit is unacceptable.

Let A Thin Person Be Your Role Model

Watching thin people can inspire us to change our behavior in other ways, too. The next time you're at a buffet, be it a wedding or a dinner out, observe the types and amounts of food that the thin people put on their plates. Contrast that to the plates of those people there that are obviously overweight. I think you will have another visual clue about how thinking thin can help you become thin.

This tactic was recently demonstrated to me on a cruise. My skinny husband (more on him later) and I found ourselves eating dinner at an hour much earlier than we were used to. We generally have dinner between 8 and 9 PM. Here we were eating at 6:30 PM. Since we weren't truly famished when we sat down to dinner, we didn't overeat too much.

But other people were ordering incredible amounts of food! On a cruise you can order whatever you want in whatever quantity. For instance, you can order an appetizer, a soup, a salad, an entrée with two side dishes, and dessert; and you can have two of everything if you want it. We seldom ordered an appetizer or a soup, although I must admit that when we did they were scrumptious. We always had a salad, an entrée, and a dessert on most nights. With that much food I gained two pounds in the week. Imagine the damage I could have done if I had ordered each and every course!

It was interesting to watch what other people ordered. The thinner cruisers stuck to salads and entrees while the heavier people indulged in every form of treat. Furthermore, the heavier folks also ate heavy breakfasts and lunches and tended to lounge by the pool.

Breakfast was an especially telling time. I would personally rather eat breakfast than any other meal of the day so I was loading up on eggs and bacon and all the things I usually avoid. Honestly, I felt guilty. I knew exactly the mistakes I was making in my food selections and I really didn't care at that point. But because I felt guilt, I found myself watching the thinner passengers with more scrutiny. Most of the thin women glided by my table with yogurt and fruit or cereal or oatmeal. Their choices were indicative of their body size in every instance. Except for mine! I was definitely on a vacation from weight control!

Lunch afforded another opportunity to watch and learn from the thinner people on board. Again, most heavy people loaded up on pizza and pasta entrees. Most thin people had salads. I was one of the salad eaters, but I made up for it by grabbing a luscious dessert...for lunch! How decadent can you get?

You can observe these same behaviors at any restaurant, particularly buffets. Watch and see what people eat and the quantities they consume. If we learn to emulate the behaviors of thin people we can often become thinner ourselves.

People complain to me all the time that their thin friends can eat anything they want. I hear tales of lunches where the thin people drink copious quantities of beer and consume every fat-laden treat on the menu, particularly nachos and potato skins. (Apparently nachos and potato skins are two items we dieters covet. The beer is a close second!)

I have to admit that this phenomenon does occur. It's not so evident in the cruise settings because you can see the "thin behavior" over a longer term. Thin people will, however, overindulge at just one meal. And it may well be the one meal you are sharing with them. Just please believe me when I tell you they would not be thin if they didn't compensate for that meal over a period of time. They may compensate through exercise or by exhibiting certain eating behaviors.

Thin People Move More

Most of the people in the cruise ship gym were thin, and all of the ones I saw routinely jogging or walking also fell into that category. The people on the rock wall and the basketball court, and those whizzing around on roller blades, were trim and fit. Contrast that to those people lounging by the pool and "bellying up" to the bar and you see my point. Likewise, thin people eat more nutritious foods in smaller quantities.

Since there's always an exception to every rule, I have to point out my own husband's behavior. He is very thin and always has been. I don't think I have weighed less than him except on our wedding day. His diet is heinous. His nutrition is abominable. He eats and drinks all the things I cannot have. Being around him day in and day out is a test of my will and determination to control my weight. It's just a good thing I love him with all my heart!

His personal weight control behavior is one I could never imitate because I cannot eat just a small portion of my trigger foods and be satisfied. I would have to eat the whole jar of peanut butter rather than just a tablespoon. Actually, I could eat just one tablespoon but fifteen minutes later I'd be going back for more, and fifteen minutes after that I'd have two tablespoons, and so on and so on until the entire jar was finished.

Thin People Prioritize Their Food Choices

Some successful dieters, the ones with less compulsive personalities, do find that they can have small amounts of fatty, calorie-laden foods and be satisfied. One such person said this to me once, but in a very succinct way. I asked Louise, who had lost a great deal of weight and was close to her goal, what her best advice would be to someone just beginning the weight loss process. I remember she was quite thoughtful for a moment and then said, "I only eat the foods I really love now."

That was a revelation to me. I asked her to expound.

"Well, I used to eat everything and anything, but now I prioritize my food choices. I now think long and hard about what I really want to eat and then I have a small amount. Before, I would eat around and around the foods I truly enjoyed because I thought they were taboo. Now I know I can eat what I want most as long as I eat smaller portions."

I immediately thought of my husband. He picks and chooses his indulgences. I knew that tactic was not one I could incorporate into my life, but it may be one you can use in yours.

It isn't surprising to me anymore to find that many, many overweight women have very thin husbands who generally can eat whatever they want, whenever they want. I admire these ladies for their compunction since they are always surrounded by behavior and food that they cannot indulge in themselves. It's a very difficult situation.

That said, I have to say that despite the poor food choices my husband makes, he eats like a bird. His portions are usually quite small. He also does not eat out of stress. Actually, stressful situations cause him not to eat at all. He does not exercise, per se. His job is sedentary, but when he is off from work he is always on his feet, busy doing, doing, doing. I don't recommend his diet or his behavior, but I use it to illustrate that even though he eats the wrong foods, he stays thin by eating very small portions. I worry about his nutrition because I know he cannot be taking in the nutrients his body requires, but I can only do (and nag) so much. The rest is up to him.

If you, too, are living with a thin husband, take heart in knowing you are not alone. You have lots of company and many compatriots. Remember Jack Sprat and his wife. They were the perfect couple. To the rest of you, listen, watch, and learn from the thin people around you. Think thin and you will be thin! Think about yourself before you sacrifice your well-being for others and you will be healthier, happier, and more fun to be around.

Things to remember from this chapter:

- Effective time management is an essential tool for weight management. Learn it well.

- You cannot please all of the people all of the time and still be sane and fit. The better motto would be: After me, you come first. Take care of yourself and then you will be able to take care of others.

- Emulate a thin person. Do what they do. Think of yourself as already being thin and exhibiting thin behaviors.

- Move more.

- Prioritize your food choices. Eat only what you really, really want; and eat it in small portions.

Chapter 8 – You Gotta Have A Goal

A goal weight is defined as the final weight you wish to learn to maintain. It may not be the weight you wish to maintain for the rest of your life, but it is where you want to be for the foreseeable future. Sometimes it's a good idea to lose a chunk of weight, learn how to maintain the loss, and then lose some more.

Reaching your weight goal is the culmination of events and efforts that begin small but mount up to great success. Your first mission is to lose 5 pounds. Your second mission is to lose 10 pounds. Then you focus on losing 10% of your starting weight. If you started out weighting 175 pounds, your 10% goal would be 17 ½ pounds.

The rationale for these goals is two-fold: first, you need something to shoot for that seems attainable, and second, after losing 10% of your body weight, you begin to enjoy numerous health benefits. Generally speaking, losing 10% of your body weight causes blood pressure to decrease, cholesterol levels to drop, weight strain on joints to decrease, and energy levels to skyrocket.

Some people may not need to lose so much weight. For them, their first or second goal may be their goal weight. Lucky them!

Choosing A Goal Weight

Thinking about your ideal weight can be very revealing. Some people envision themselves at their lowest weight ever. Others want to weigh what they weighed when they graduated from high school or college, or when they got married. All these time references are very popular with dieters. Sometimes those weights are attainable and desirable, but more often than not they are just a fond memory.

"That was then and this is now," I like to say. When there are thirty years between then and now, the weight goal in mind just might be unrealistic. And an unrealistic weight goal can be a very disturbing thing. Inability to maintain the weight loss, or finding that it takes too much time and effort to maintain that goal, is not uncommon.

Honestly answering several questions will help you arrive at a comfortable goal.

- How hard or easy has it been to lose the weight to this point?

- How much time and effort are you devoting to the effort to lose the weight?

- Why have you chosen this particular number (weight goal)?

- Are you happy with the way you look and feel?

Your initial weight goal chosen is merely a target. It is not written in stone and can be changed at any time. The decision is always yours. Sometimes, however, an independent observer's opinion is important. As an outside observer may have a better perspective than the person who is wholly consumed with the effort and the achievement of weight loss.

As a matter of illustration, let's take a look at Jane's situation. She has maintained a weight loss of about fifteen pounds for over 21 years. She is very slim and her goal weight is at the low end of her weight range for her height and age. In fact, the upper limits of those ranges expand with age, so she is even further away from the upper end of the range than she was when she initially lost weight. All these years she has worked to stay at this weight and when I say "worked," I mean it!

Recently she's had trouble keeping her weight down. A one or two pound gain for her is the end of the world, mind you! After all those years of "watching it" she met a motivational lag that troubled her deeply. I saw her in tears over this situation. My advice to her was to jump start her exercise program because she had been walking three miles most days all those years.

The problem with that routine is that doing it so religiously means that the body adapts to that stress and the workout becomes less and less challenging over time. I asked her to intersperse some light jogging into her routine and it worked like magic. Suddenly she lost the few pounds that plagued her and she renewed her motivation at the same time.

I still worry about her because she allows herself almost no indulgences at all. While understanding her feeling that if she gives herself an inch, she'll take a mile, I also see where her life is very restrictive and her regime very demanding. As she ages, she may be faced with having to raise her goal weight to a level she can live with and I fear that will be a big hurdle for her. Her identity and self-worth are too intimately related to the numbers on the scale!

Goal Weights Can Fluctuate

Goal weights are meant to fluctuate with changing life situations. I, myself, found that my initial goal weight required much too much effort to maintain so I raised it by ten pounds seven years after making goal. In my opinion, as long as your weight is no more than ten pounds above the maximum weight range for your height, you are fine. The ranges at the website noted below seem restrictive to me, but they provide a guideline and a "best case scenario."

Weight ranges change periodically as medical recommendations are made about what constitutes a healthy weight. The ranges are usually the same ones that insurance companies refer to when determining someone's health risk from their weight. The Rush University Medical Center publishes an ideal height/weight range table, and it may be found at the following website: http://www.rush.edu/rumc/page-1108048103230.html. The weight ranges are for guidance only. Do not become discouraged if you don't "measure up."

Sometimes life circumstances demand that we adapt. Adapting and giving up are two entirely different things! An illness or injury may require a goal weight adjustment, but you should look at it that way. Do not see an opportunity to backslide. Knowing that goals are flexible should be comforting as you struggle to get to your final "magic number."

Another client who comes to mind is Galene. She was relatively slim when she asked me to coach her, but was absolutely determined to lose weight. She worked very hard and even took up running to lose her 10% and more. Now she is seven pounds above the minimum weight for her height and age and she wants to lose those last seven pounds. The problem is she's hungry.

"I don't know why but I'm hungry all the time, Sue. What am I doing wrong?" she asks.

I methodically go through all the possibilities including her not eating enough, to not eating enough protein or fat, to not drinking enough water and she assures me she is doing all those vital things. I tell her I will think about the problem when she says, "I even tried not running one week thinking that maybe the running was making me too hungry. That week I gained a whole pound!"

I pondered the situation for a while and then suggested that she be happy with her weight right where it is. Losing those extra seven pounds will probably only make her hungrier, and if she's hungry at this weight, imagine how difficult maintaining that seven pound loss will be. I can't say yet what her reaction to that suggestion might be, but I bet it isn't positive. People have certain number goals stuck in their heads and even in the face of mounting evidence that the goal is unrealistic, the appeal of those numbers continues to shine. Remember that reaching goal weight is one thing. Maintaining that goal weight is quite another.

Unrealistic Goals

Sometimes people who far below their goal weights. I worry that they'll slip from one extreme to another and fall into the anorexia trap. Having such control over their food intake may be an entirely new feeling for them. And in some instances that control can seem like the only control one has over their life, especially when things get chaotic. Anorexia is at its heart a control issue.

Don't struggle to maintain an unrealistic goal weight. It can zap your energy and self-esteem and may ultimately backfire, causing you to give up the struggle completely. Do what you can with what you've got and enjoy your success.

Goal Weights For Men

Goal weights may even be outside the ranges, as long as they are not lower than what is suitable for your age and height. A weight above the range is acceptable to me as long as it is acceptable to you. Men, in particular, cringe when they see the goal weight ranges. I'd love to have a dollar for each time I've heard an incredulous man say to me, "What?! I didn't even weight that in high school!!" I usually want to respond by saying, "Well you should have weighed that in high school!"

No distinction is made these days between weight ranges established for men and women. Years ago, men were given much more leeway but no more. A healthy weight is determined by your height and age alone. (I'd also like to have a dollar for each time a five-foot tall woman has told me she's really 6'2"!)

I think men sometimes balk at the idea of losing below 200 pounds because they have an artificial block at that level. Perhaps it's because the weight becomes harder to lose the lighter you become and they think crossing the two hundred pound threshold will make the process too difficult. Perhaps they've never weighed less than 200 and think they can't do it now.

Whatever the reason, many men choose a goal weight outside of the normal ranges only to meet that goal and keep losing down to a weight within the range. Somehow that magical 200 number relieves their pressure to succeed and men in particular seem to need that relief in order to get to goal. I can't explain the psychological basis for the phenomenon but I see it all the time.

One man was convinced that he had lost enough weight after dropping thirty pounds. He held this conviction despite the fact that he was 5'8" and weighed over 200. His wife even took a picture of him to convince him that he still had more weight to lose. This picture apparently showed more of him than he would have liked because he told me it was the picture that kept him going. He hasn't made much progress beyond the thirty pounds but he has kept that weight off for a year or more. Perhaps a photo really should be taken to help determine a person's goal weight.

Short-Term Goals

From mid-March to June is when people develop short-term goals. There are June brides, June mothers-of-the-bride (or groom), June graduates, June "I need to wear a swimsuit - GASP!"-vacationers, among others. Their goals are not necessarily long-term; their goals may be to drop 20 pounds in ten weeks!

The problem is that losing weight in such a manner provides no incentive for keeping it off. The example that comes to mind is one that knocked me for a loop. A wonderful woman named Kathy made wonderful strides in improving her diet and nutrition and losing weight, too. This lady is an accomplished educator and a bonafide overachiever, so it didn't surprise me that she was always on track. In the course of six months she lost over 35 pounds and completely transformed herself. Her success was a beautiful thing to watch as she blossomed and her attire began to reflect the new Kathy. Stylish outfits replaced the baggy garments she wore before her weight loss and her skirts grew shorter and shorter as her thighs grew slimmer and slimmer.

She reached maintenance and suddenly lost her focus. In maintenance, it is extremely important to closely monitor food intake to find out "what you can get away with." You need to establish the uppermost limits of your food intake without gaining weight. To do this you must chronicle food intake closely. Kathy wouldn't do it. My overachiever became a slacker overnight!

Weeks went by and it became obvious she was gaining the weight back. I'd try talking to her but never got a satisfactory explanation for her actions. Then one day we talked.

"Kathy, what is going on with you?" I asked.

"I'm just not doing it anymore," she responded.

"Have you just lost your focus?"

That's when she knocked me for a loop. "As soon as the occasion was over I lost all my motivation."

"The occasion?" I inquired, very much surprised.

"Yeah, I had something I had to attend and that was my goal, to lose weight for that occasion."

Suddenly her struggles all made perfect sense to me. "Oh!" I said. "I had no idea that there was a goal other than a weight goal. Then you succeeded in doing what you set out to do. No wonder you're having such trouble now."

She looked at me, puzzled. "You need to refocus your goal now," I explained. "The goal you had is passed and you need to make a decision to reach this weight goal for YOU. Not for an occasion, or for anyone else. It has to be for you now."

I'm sure she understood, but she apparently couldn't make that switch. Her desire to keep the weight off was not great enough to motivate her after her special occasion passed. I mourn the stylish new outfits hanging in her closet unworn. The example, however, is an important one to understand as you make your way to your weight goal.

Goals Need To Be Specific

Goals are equally important at every phase of your weight loss journey. The important thing is to make them specific.

Ask someone why they are dieting.

Invariably they reply, "To lose weight!"

"Okay, then. If you lose one pound over a three week period you'll be happy, right?"

With boos and groans they answer, "NO!"

"Well why not," I ask. "You said you wanted to lose weight and you did. How can you argue with that?"

"That's not enough weight for three weeks," everyone says.

Which is exactly my point. The goal was not specific enough. Saying you want to lose one to two pounds a week for ten weeks is specific enough to motivate you. Adding specifics make the goal attainable. Then you can know when you have succeeded and when you haven't. But is one to two pounds a week fast enough? It should be enough because that is a healthy amount of weight to lose each week. Slow and Steady wins the race.

Things to remember from this chapter:

- You have to set smaller, specific, attainable goals in the beginning of your weight loss journey.

- Ask yourself specific questions to set your final goal weight. Question your reasoning for choosing that particular number on the scale.

- Keep maintenance in mind.

- Be gentle with yourself

Chapter 9 - Motivation

All that goal setting is designed to motivate you to start, continue, and persevere until you get where you are going. Setting attainable, specific goals is one of the best ways to motivate yourself to lose the weight and keep it off. The problem is that motivation is a thing that comes and goes, waxes and wanes. It is not static or constant, but instead it is constantly changing. The reasons for the change can be anything from your health to your results, to your emotional well-being. Motivation for anything, but especially weight loss, is a very individual thing.

Over the years the most often asked question is, "How can I get back the motivation I had before?"

I always respond by sighing and saying, "I wish I could just throw the switch that would make you gung-ho to get to your weight goal. If I had that magic wand, I would use it on you, and everyone else. Of course, I'd have to charge you for it and then I'd go live the rest of my life in a beach house in Fiji."

The Stages Of Motivation

In the early stages of weight loss people are generally thoroughly "pumped" to conquer the problem and embark on a new journey of healthy living. They sometimes, not always, but sometimes, have already talked themselves into the necessity of weight loss and are eager to get started.

Over time, though, that motivation naturally wanes. In fact, professionals categorize the weight loss journey into four distinct periods, all reflecting differing levels of motivation. These phases are equally applicable to any effort at behavior modification be it weight control, smoking cessation, or drug addiction counseling.

The Stages Of Motivation: Phase 1

The first phase in the effort is known as the Honeymoon, or "Let Me At It" Phase. This is when you are reading every last bit of nutrition and weight loss material that you can get your hands on. You scrutinize nutrition labels until you have everything you eat regularly committed to memory. Then you subscribe to various health and fitness publications which serve to further motivate you.

Every morsel you eat is scrutinized, sometimes even weighed, and you write down everything you eat. Not one thing is missing. Even portions are shown and accounted for in writing. Generally a new exercise commitment accompanies your new-found interest in healthy eating.

During this phase, weight loss comes relatively quickly and easily. Each loss serves to further reinforce the new behaviors and motivates you to continue the effort. Hopefully, this phase lasts a good long time. It can actually last the entire time until you meet your weight goal, and aren't you lucky if it does!

The Stages Of Motivation: Phase 2

Unfortunately, though, for most people the second phase intervenes. I call this time period the Honeymoon Is Over phase (or the Plateau). Generally speaking, after losing twenty pounds or so, it is common to enter a plateau period where you adhere to your behavior but see no more weight loss. There are several reasons for this experience.

The first is that you may not be adhering to those behaviors as strictly as you think you are. Upon questioning, most people will admit that they have grown somewhat complacent during this period. Their food diaries are not as complete as they used to be. They are not being as strict with their portions. Many times I'll ask, "Are you still eating the same foods in the same amounts that you were eating before?"

Looking at their feet and shuffling a bit, the response will be, "I think so."

"You think so? What does that mean?" I ask.

"Well, I'm not sure. I'm not paying attention like I was before."

Is that what Oprah calls an Ah-Ha moment? It's certainly revealing.

This phase is when we feel proud of ourselves for losing the twenty pounds and we decide to reward ourselves with an extra glass of wine or an extra portion of mashed potatoes. It's also when we come to really crave whatever favorite foods we have gone without for the past several months. If we feel deprived because we haven't tasted our favorites for a long time, there is a danger of overeating now that wasn't necessarily a danger in the Honeymoon Phase.

Recognizing these behaviors is the first step in reining them in. Being twenty pounds lighter also means that you are not expending as many calories through exercise as you were at a heavier weight. That's not an obvious fact, but it's one to think about.

Walking a mile carrying 195 pounds is going to be more strenuous than walking a mile carrying 175 pounds, right? So now you might need to walk a mile and a half to burn the same number of calories you were burning when you first started your weight loss journey.

This phase is just that.....another phase. Knowing that everyone, or most everyone, goes through the same challenging times on their way to success may help spur you on to Phase 3.

The Stages Of Motivation: Phase 3

And Phase 3 is where you recommit yourself to your initial healthy behaviors and regain the determination you first had to succeed. Many things can help get you from Phase 2 to Phase 3.

Tactics To Get From Phase 2 To Phase 3

One is reading the success stories of others. Most health and fitness magazines contain a section on Success Stories. These articles are usually the most popular ones in the entire magazine. People tend to turn to these testimonials first, before reading anything else. Why? Because these are real people and they give us the motivation to get to our goals. If they can do it then we can do it. These real folks don't have the benefit of celebrity personal trainers and personal chefs and personal secretaries. They have the same everyday headaches and chores and tasks that we have, and they succeeded anyway.

Join the "Win When You Lose" Facebook page. Interact with others and take your cues from them. I'll be there, too, to urge you on and applaud your efforts. Sometimes a gentle nudge is all you need to get from Phase 2 to Phase 3.

Yet another path from Phase 2 to newfound commitment in Phase 3 might be to try on some of the clothes you were wearing when you first began to lose weight. The adage that a picture is worth a thousand words is true. Look at yourself in the mirror as you swim around in your old clothes and think how much better you look and feel at your new weight. Likewise, perusing the old photo album and seeing the "before" you sometimes helps kick start a stalled weight loss effort.

In fact, I've had clients who thought they were comfortable at their present weight look at a recent photograph and decide it was time to start anew. They were not where they wanted to be yet in terms of their appearance. You would think that looking in a mirror would have the same effect, but don't fool yourself into thinking that it does. I can't explain why, but you can somehow imagine yourself a lot thinner than you actually are when you look into a mirror. It's as though you see what you want to see rather than what's really there. A photograph has a much more "slap in the face" type of effect.

The Stages Of Motivation: Phase 4...Finally

So you survive the challenge of Phase 2 and find yourself recommitted to your efforts in Phase 3. That's wonderful! Because this is where you will alter your behavior to get the results you need and you will eventually reach your final weight goal. Sometime during this phase you may find yourself adhering to the regime you have set for yourself as a matter of course. Those healthy behaviors become second nature at this point.

When you slip into that mode of operation you have achieved Phase 4, known as Changed Lifestyle. This is when your weight loss efforts shift from being a "diet" or behavior specifically geared towards weight loss. Instead, you behave in such a way as to support the new you.

You find yourself making healthy choices because they suit your lifestyle and make you feel good, not merely because they help you maintain your weight or lose pounds. This Phase is the ultimate success. It's where you come to believe that you are in fact a new person with new values and new aspirations.

Not every person who embarks on the weight loss journey makes it to this point. Very few do, really. So embrace the moment and the feeling of accomplishment. Hard work and perseverance got you to this point and you fully deserve all the good things that come your way. Congratulations!

Things to remember from this chapter:

Motivation

- Motivation comes and goes in fits and starts.

- There are methods you can use to recapture your motivation when it wanes.

- There are four stages of motivation when you are trying to kick a bad habit. Recognize the stages and understand how to progress from one to another.

- A picture of yourself can be a very motivating tool.

Chapter 10 – Slow And Steady Wins The Weight Loss Race

How do you define "success?" Is it losing 20 pounds? Is getting to your goal weight and maintaining it for a year? Maybe success is maintaining the weight loss for several years. For weight loss, though, slow and steady is the name of the game.

Losing one to two pounds per week is the standard weight loss rate considered healthy. It is not a "quick fix." Slow weight loss, however, promotes lifestyle and habit changes. Over the course of time, you will be able to learn what you need to learn and make the eating and lifestyle changes habit. Steady, moderately paced weight loss is the name of this game.

Is That All I Lost?

That kind of slow, steady progress is not what most people want.

Take Marina, for instance. She isn't too heavy, maybe she's fifteen pounds overweight. She expressed her concern that she had turned 40 years old and figured there was no way to trim down at that advanced age. She felt her fate was sealed until she read some testimonials from similarly aged women on various internet sites. Those testimonials gave her hope and motivated her to look for a weight loss solution.

After a week, I casually passed by and asked, "So how'd you do your first week, Marina?"

I was shocked when she looked up, obviously distressed, with her eyes welling up with tears.

"I lost a little, she sniffed.

"How much is 'a little'?"

"A pound and a half," she said dejectedly.

"That's PERFECT!" I responded. "So why are you upset?"

"I thought I'd lose more," she said with a sigh.

"Well, I'm sorry you're disappointed but you have to remember that one to two pounds a week is a healthy weight loss. It is all you should expect."

"Really?" She seemed to straighten up a little and a hopeful look returned to her face.

"Yes! You did a great job! You realize a slower loss is more likely to stay off, right?"

"I know that," she said. "I guess I didn't put all this weight on at once so I can't expect to take it off at once, either."

That conversation helped spur Marina on to lose another two pounds the following week. It seems no matter how many times I remind people that one to two pounds of weight loss each week is a good thing, I always hear, "Oh, I only lost a pound this week...." That amounts to 52 pounds a year - and who in their right mind wouldn't be happy with that?

As a footnote, I think Marina's unrealistic expectations stayed with her and prevented her from succeeding. She lost several more pounds over the next few weeks, and then told me she was going out of town for two weeks on a business trip. I never saw her again.

Any Try Is A Good Try

Even these relatively short-lived attempts at weight loss have their rewards, despite what the popular press would have you believe. The popular theory right now is that efforts to lose weight are actually unhealthy. This thought process certainly helps us all evade the weight problem and pat ourselves on the back for not even trying. The problem is that it just isn't true. Any effort is better than no effort at all, provided it's healthy.

Many times people take some small behavior change away from each weight loss attempt. Maybe they continue to drink eight glasses of water every day. Maybe they eat more fruits and vegetables. Perhaps they read nutrition labels more often. All of these little positive changes can come together at a later date to form the framework that makes long-term weight loss and maintenance a reality. No one should ever feel that an effort "failed." There is always some positive aspect to each "try." As stated in the beginning of this book, dieting efforts should be applauded and never viewed as failures. They are good tries, always.

In fact, I'm sometimes glad to hear people say they've tried to lose weight before because it means they've learned something in that effort. Now we just have to build on and reinforce what they learned.

I am not so happy to hear people say they have tried a get-thin-quick program. A former colleague used to say "diet" stands for Did I Eat Today? In most cases, the answer is, "No!" Not eating can cause more problems than it solves. It is not the answer to weight loss. The get-thin-quick programs usually involve starvation. We'll see in the next chapter why this method is so counterproductive.

Everyone Loses Weight Differently

Some people regard their slow weight loss as a kind of failure. Please understand that everyone loses weight at different rates. When other people are losing several pounds a week, it can make you feel like an underachiever to lose half a pound. The truth of the matter is that some people are just built that way. Everyone is different, even at weight loss. Metabolisms vary, as do activity levels, ages, sex, and a multitude of other variables that dictate how fast you can lose a pound of fat.

Slow And Steady Wins The Weight Loss Race

Everyone needs to remember that this is not a contest or a competition. If you happen to be the one struggling to lose 1/2 a pound a week and you see someone lose five pounds in their first effort, it can be discouraging. Fast weight loss does not necessarily mean permanent weight loss, and in fact generally the faster you lose the faster you gain it all back. Losing fast doesn't give your habits and lifestyle a chance to change along with your body and without those changes you are on the diet rollercoaster forever.

Sharon writes to me in a personal e-mail: "And losing a pound over a few weeks is nothing compared to everyone else, while I'm grateful I didn't gain. I don't know why it is such a hard struggle for me to lose maybe half a pound a week when others lose pounds. I think that's why I get discouraged with myself."

The key word in that note is "compared." When she compares herself to everyone else is when she gets discouraged. I understand the desire to compete and compare is innate, however, it can be detrimental to your weight loss efforts. I also understand how hard it is to stay motivated when you lose weight slowly.

My husband calls me an "air plant." I hardly need food at all to survive and can gain weight eating only a little bit over subsistence levels. I understand totally how slow losers feel. The lady in the example above has now lost over 24 pounds as those half-pounds have mounted up. Slow and steady wins the weight loss race!

Things to remember from this chapter:

- You should aim to lose one to two pounds a week. This amounts to 52 to 104 pounds in a year!

- You learn something with every effort at weight loss. No effort is ever a failure.

- Never compare your weight loss experience to anyone else's.

- Slow and steady weight losses are the ones that are maintained over time.

Chapter 11 – Staying Satisfied

How are you going to embark on this process and not suffer? Simple answer: You are not going to let yourself get too hungry.

Planning Is Everything

Weight management is one of those things that require proper planning. There's no getting around it. From your grocery list to meal planning and preparation to knowing what foods keep you satisfied longest, planning is everything. I'm not sure to whom I should attribute this quote but I use it all the time: "Fail to plan and you plan to fail."

You know that if you come home from work starving you throw open the refrigerator and the pantry and the cabinets and begin to randomly devour whatever you find there. It doesn't matter what it is, but I can bet you it won't be carrots and low-fat yogurt! Chances are you'll reach for something that will give you an immediate boost: something like pretzels or crackers with maybe some cheese and peanut butter thrown in for good measure. Do you know why you do that?

Those pretzels and crackers are called refined carbohydrates. That means they have been processed so that most of the fiber has been removed. When you eat these types of foods, your blood insulin level goes sky high in short order. That's the immediate boost of energy you feel. The problem is, those foods are digested very quickly, leaving you with that high insulin level in your bloodstream which compels you to eat more because you remain hungry. This explains why one handful of pretzels is seldom enough and you end up going back for more, and more. Eating refined carbohydrates when you are very hungry creates a Catch-22 or vicious cycle situation that leads to overeating.

The cheese and the peanut butter, however, are heavy on fat and protein; both of these nutrients take longer to digest and make you feel satisfied. The problem with these is that you don't get the immediate feeling of having eaten something because they take longer for your body to process. Many times you'll end up eating too much cheese or peanut butter before that feeling of satiety kicks in. Of course, low-fat cheese and low-fat peanut butter will have less of a detrimental effect on your weight by virtue of their (presumably) lower calorie count.

Perhaps the best choice under these ravenous circumstances (and you should never come home this ravenous anyway because you should have planned your eating better throughout the day) would be a whole grain product that takes longer to digest but doesn't take as long as the fat and protein. It won't spike your insulin level to the extent refined carbohydrates do. A bowl of oatmeal, a low-fat bran muffin, or some whole wheat bread are all good suggestions. Low fat Greek yogurt is also a good choice for its mix of protein and low-carbohydrates. The key is to understand how different foods and nutrients affect your feeling of satisfaction and to use each in the appropriate circumstance.

Everyone is different, though. Some people tend towards eating more carbohydrates than protein and others go the other way towards more protein. If you've never thought about it, you may not know exactly what your tendency is so be aware of how food works for you. If you are feeling hungry by mid-morning, you might want to switch your cereal and milk at breakfast for an egg white omelet. The protein may be more satisfying to you. It might not. You need to experiment to find out.

As far as I'm concerned, it's really up to you what you eat when. You are smart enough to know what foods support your weight loss efforts and which don't. You can also just choose any diet you feel comfortable with. It makes no difference which one you use, really. It's staying on it that is difficult, and that's what this book tries to help you with.

I will tell you that you should not drink your calories. Soda, fruit juices, full-sugar flavored waters, high-calorie energy drinks, will all ruin your diet and set you up to be hungry, too. The quick sugar rush (energy) that you feel raises your insulin level and later leaves you famished. Plus, the calories mount up. Eat an orange instead of drinking OJ. Eat some peanut butter crackers with a diet soda. Have a low-fat string cheese with your no-sugar water. Now that's how to stay satisfied.

Don't think breakfast has to be traditional, either. I have a friend who is a Physician's Assistant and never gets to lunch before 3 PM. Her solution is to eat a low-fat meat and cheese sandwich on the way to work because she knows that will keep her energy levels up until her late lunchtime rolls around. She has lost over 50 pounds and has maintained that loss through all kinds of lifestyle upheavals, so take note of her problem-solving techniques. Meals don't have to be traditional. They just have to keep you satisfied.

Same Old Advice: Eat Breakfast!

Eating breakfast has always been an unwritten rule in the annuals of weight loss history. I can't think of one diet I have been on, and I've been on most of them for thirty years, that didn't advise you to eat breakfast. It's a good habit to get into. When I suggest people eat breakfast their reply is often, "If I don't eat, I don't get hungry and then I can wait until one o'clock before I have lunch. Eating breakfast makes me hungry and then I have to have something by 11 AM."

Let's analyze this situation. If you are not getting hungry until half of the day has elapsed, then your metabolism has never started running. It's like a car engine. You have to give it fuel to make it run. Feeling hunger is a GOOD thing. It means you are burning calories. Hunger is not the enemy just as food is not the enemy. Both are your allies in the weight war. You just need to know how to use them productively.

By eating something, anything, in the morning (just a slice of toast may be enough) you are activating your engine to run and burn either fat or glucose as fuel. This is a desirable thing. Because it causes you to eat a snack at 11 AM does not mean you will gain weight. Quite the contrary, what you have eaten at breakfast and mid-morning will be burned off PLUS MORE. Not eating and not getting hungry means you have not started the engine and have burned no fuel for more than half of your day. You cannot lose weight that way. You need to maximize the calorie burning potential of your body all day long. And you need to stay satisfied as well. Breakfast can help you in both respects. There's more information on this topic in the following Chapter titled, "You Have To Eat To Lose."

Eat What You Want Or Else You Will Eat Around It

Sometimes you just don't know what you want. Or do you? A longtime client at her goal weight recounted a Christmas evening. "Someone sent us a fruitcake and it was sitting on the kitchen counter. I was watching TV but all I could think of was 'I want some fruitcake' so I went into the kitchen and ate a tangerine. I was still hungry. So I ate some bread. Then I went back into the living room and started watching TV again and I was thinking 'I really want that fruitcake' so I went back into the kitchen and ate the fruitcake. So I ended up eating the tangerine, the bread, AND the damned fruitcake when I could have just had the fruitcake!!" Sally is very refreshing in her candid remarks. She often speaks of situations we have all been in but have neglected to SEE.

I call this eating around what you really want. It is counter-productive, so eat what you really want in a normal portion. If the desired food is a trigger food, then have it in a controlled situation, say at a restaurant where the portion is limited.

I vividly recall a conversation that turned into one of the funniest I have ever enjoyed. We brainstormed some suggestions about staying satisfied, many of which had a psychological component, such as staying focused on your goal and deriving satisfaction from that, and thinking that the first bite of any food is "tasting" and subsequent bites are "eating." (I thought that comment was very insightful.)

At any rate, I meant to wrap up the topic by saying, "So play mind games with yourself.." and instead ended up saying, "So play with yourselves..." There was a deafening silence as everyone took that comment in and suddenly someone loudly asked, "So how many calories can you spend doing that?" Laughter erupted everywhere and one of my helpers, Sarah, stepped forward and said, 'I was just reading where you burn 100 calories in 30 minutes having sex."

I thought for a moment and said, "Well then you aren't doing it right."

Another woman asked, "Sarah, where did you read that?"

"I just read it in my AARP magazine."

There was a murmur in the audience and someone said, "Well THAT explains it!" More laughter ensued and I knew I had lost control

The rest of the evening was lost to riotous laughter and bawdy humor but everyone definitely went home with a smile on their faces. The Staying Satisfied message would be remembered.

Things to remember from this chapter:

- Proper planning is essential to weight loss. Plan your meals, your shopping, your indulgences, your everything.

- Know and notice the effect different kinds of foods (fats, protein, whole grains, refined carbohydrates) have on your body. Choose your food types wisely according to what foods keep you satisfied longest.

- Eat breakfast to stoke your furnace.

- If you want something, eat it. Don't eat AROUND it!

- Have fun wherever and whenever you can.

- You don't have to suffer and starve to lose weight. Keep yourself satisfied!

- The first bite of every food is "tasting," but subsequent bites are "eating".

Chapter 12 – You Have To Eat To Lose

You cannot starve yourself thin. You can if you have an eating disorder like anorexia, but otherwise, forget it. You don't need to starve yourself to lose weight, anyway, and you don't need to exercise excessively, either.

The Body Is Efficient

The body is a very efficient machine. If you starve it, it will fight to hold onto every ounce of energy it has and will actually lower your metabolism to conserve its energy (fat) stores. A slower metabolism makes it much harder to lose weight so the end result of eating too little is that you are starving and yet not losing an ounce.

Now, the heavier you are, the more food and calories you need just to move around. A heavier person will likewise expend more energy at whatever activity they undertake.

Unfortunately, that means the slimmer you get, the less food you can eat and still maintain your weight loss. You either have to increase your exercise or cut back on your calories. This cutback usually naturally occurs as you lose weight, so don't worry about it now.

Just recently I met an older blond woman who looked very suspicious when I mentioned that you had to eat enough food to keep your metabolism running and to lose weight. I intuitively knew there was an issue to address.

"Diana," I asked, "do you have a problem with that?"

There was a long silent pause and she said, "I don't eat that much."

I launched into my spiel and she immediately got a glazed look in her eyes. It was obvious that I had lost her.

You Have To Eat To Lose

I sighed, "You don't believe what I'm telling you, do you?"

That's when another woman piped up and said, "That happened to me. I wasn't eating enough to lose weight and Sue and I talked and she told me I had to eat more. I was skeptical but your body is like a car or a furnace. You have to give it fuel to make it run and if you don't, it will just sit there and conserve whatever fuel it has. You can't lose weight like that."

I could see Diana was accepting this as fact.

Many weeks later I asked if there were any surprises that anyone had experienced recently and Diana responded without hesitation.

"I was surprised I could eat so much food and still lose weight," she said.

"I remember our first conversation. You didn't believe that to be true at all," I said.

"No, I didn't believe it when you said it, but when that other lady told me, then I decided it was probably true."

I didn't question her much further about why she didn't believe me but did believe the other lady. She probably wouldn't have had an answer, anyway. The good thing is that the two helped one another and she got the message and lost weight. Without accepting the fact that you have to eat to lose, Diana would have starved herself, not lost any weight, and walked away unhappy with me and even more sadly, unhappy with herself.

Many, many of the most overweight people I encounter actually eat very little. They obviously ate a lot in the past to become so obese, but at a later date they can eat like birds and remain morbidly obese because of the metabolism's adaptation described above.

Food Is Not The Enemy

It's a challenge to get these people to understand that "you have to eat to lose." In their minds, food is the enemy. Food is why they are so uncomfortable. To convince them that they have to eat more to lose weight goes against the logic they know to be true.

Since I don't know what they were eating before I know them, I can't say if the difference is food quality or quantity. For example, they could be eating only four doughnuts in an entire day. That particular food choice is the equivalent calories of a bowl of high-fiber cereal with skim milk, a turkey breast and tomato sandwich, two big salads (or more) with no-fat Italian dressing, a baked chicken breast, broccoli, a 10-ounce baked potato, a small apple, a cup of grapes, an unlimited amount of vegetable soup, and a no-fat pudding cup as a snack! Perhaps it's just this quantity disparity that throws them, but they do have trouble eating enough to keep their metabolism working and lose weight.

The book "Volumetrics" by Barbara Rolls illustrates the equivalent quantity of food based on calories. The pictures speak to people where words don't get through. I highly recommend the visuals this book offers.

Not just obese people fall into this trap. Many time heavy exercisers do the same thing. One particularly memorable person comes to mind.

"I'm exercising three hours a day and I can't lose any weight."

"What kind of exercise are you doing?"

"I'm walking and doing weights with a trainer at the gym"

"Why are you devoting so much time to exercise?"

"So I can LOSE WEIGHT (implied was, "you moron")"

"Well, what are you eating?"

"I had a salad and a yogurt so far today." It was now 5 PM.

"Well, there's your problem, Bev. You aren't eating enough."

Bev gives me her best BLANK STARE.

"You have to eat enough to keep your metabolism going. You can't lose weight by starving. I want you to e-mail me what you eat for the next three days."

I'd see where she was only eating around 700 calories a day -- way under the recommended 1600 I had suggested. I'd call her and explain the situation. I wrote her with specific instructions and then called her yet again.

When we finally spoke she'd say, "I'd better lose this week. I've only eaten a salad all day."

AHHHHHH. It's enough to make you want to scream.

Another woman tells me she exercises three hours a day ("Why do you do that?" I ask. "Because I like it," she responds.), and hasn't lost an ounce. Could she think she can eat all she wants because she works out so much? Maybe. Will she send me her food diary so I can see what she's eating and make recommendations? No.

There are more Bev's out there than you would imagine and they're all stunned when (and if) they realize they can eat a large quantity of nutritious food, not be hungry, and lose weight, too.

Dieting Does Not Equal Deprivation

That d.i.e.t. mentality is a hard mind-set to break. After years of experience with the Grapefruit Diet, The Boiled Egg Diet,

The Cabbage Soup Diet and others, we've come to associate dieting with deprivation. And rightly so.

As youngsters, we learned we could lose five pounds in a week by "just not eating." Those positive experiences with weight loss stick with us into our later years. What doesn't stick with us is that souped-up teenage metabolism that allowed us to lose five pounds in a week by "just not eating." Things are different now. Boy, are they different! As we age the metabolism slows down and not eating simply slows it further. Gone are the don't eat-drop five pounds days. You have to eat to lose now. And don't you forget it.

Yet another example is Lucy lost her weight years ago and is now at her goal weight. What you wouldn't know by looking at her is that she has gained and lost fifty or more pounds over and over again in the ensuing years. She obviously did not learn how to maintain her weight loss in the first place.

By the time she came to me, I incorrectly assumed that she understood that you have to eat to lose weight and that losing is one process or skill and maintaining that loss is another. I was wrong to make those assumptions. As time passed, I came to understand that something was wrong with her thinking.

"So how are you doing Lucy?" I asked after she had lost 20 pounds.

"I'm doing great! The weight is coming off, but I knew it would. I've never had trouble losing weight," she replied with a smile.

The following week she initiated a conversation about setting her goal weight. I said, "Don't forget now, since you've lose so much weight you should be eating less than when you started this journey."

Immediately she responded with, "Oh, that's not a problem I've been eating about 600 calories a day anyway."

I'm sure my mouth dropped open and I heard myself let out an audible gasp.

"What?! You shouldn't be doing that!" I reprimanded her. "Haven't you been listening when I've told you the effects that type of starvation diet will have on your weight loss, not to mention your health!"

"I have to eat that level to lose weight," she said quite earnestly.

"Well if that's the case then you have to step up your exercise and put on some muscle mass to increase your metabolism," I threw back at her.

"I've been doing water aerobics, she replied.

"How long have you been doing that?"

"A long time."

"Well you're probably so used to doing that that it isn't having much effect then. You're going to want to try something new," I said.

"Like what?"

"What's wrong with walking? It's easy, it's cheap, it's handy. Have you tried walking before?"

"No," she said tentatively.

"Well you could go to the gym if that's more your style."

"No! No gym for me. That just isn't me," she replied.

"Well then try walking this week, eat regularly and nutritiously, and see what effect it has on your weight next week. Lucy, eating what you are eating is only around 600 calories a day. There's no way you can get your nutrition in that way and certainly no way you can possible keep your metabolism going."

"Oh, I've eaten 500 calories before."

I just stared at her and asked, sincerely, "How on earth can you torture and deprive yourself like that?"

I felt such compassion for her when she looked at me straight-on and I could see the desperation in her eyes when she said, "It's not easy."

The Vicious Cycle Ends Now

That's when I gently jumped on my soapbox. "You have done this so many times before. Losing the weight and gaining it back, and I want this to be the last time you struggle with it so much. Imagine being at your chosen weight and not having to "diet" and worry about your weight. You'd have so much extra energy for the other things in your life that you want and need to accomplish. That's why you have to learn to eat and you have to teach your body to function properly. If you are only eating 600 calories a day what do you suppose will happen when you go back to eating normally?"

"That's easy. I'll gain weight."

"Exactly. And that's the vicious cycle you are in and have been in for many, many years."

There's a world of people starving themselves in an effort to either speed up the weight loss process or lose weight without exercising. Extreme hunger is a torturous existence. Certainly not one you can endure for very long.

Usually we dieters are encouraged to eat as little as possible and you can see where that advice has gotten us all. We're on a roller coaster of yo-yo dieting that is discouraging and depressing and we're all getting fatter and fatter. Getting fatter and fatter is what happens when you starve yourself to lose weight. Without added exercise you are losing muscle mass rather than fat and then when you regain the weight you gain it as fat rather than lean muscle. So you can actually end up losing weight but being fatter than when you started.

By asking you to determine the upper level of your food intake where you can eat and be satisfied and still lose a pound a week, I am asking you to perhaps slow down the process in the hopes of ending the struggle in the long run.

Keeping food intake as high as possible will help you get necessary nutrition and engage your metabolism to boot. Then when you enter maintenance you will hopefully be eating at a level you can live with without feeling deprived.

- In the long run, you will preserve your metabolism and be able to live with your eating plan instead of suffer on a diet.

Not Everyone Struggles Like This: But Most Do

Bear in mind that these problems with inadequate food intake and low metabolism do not plague everyone. Some folks are blessed with a wonderfully high metabolic rate, other work hard to maintain their muscle mass to speed up their metabolisms, and others exercise vigorously through aerobic activity to make up for any natural shortfall.

That's not to say some people don't lose easier than others because they do. But it's the ones that struggle that are shining examples of determination and dedication. Arlene is the example that comes to mind. She's had her share of medical problems. Nevertheless, Arlene was losing weight steadily for perhaps eight weeks. Suddenly she stopped losing for several weeks. I attributed it to a lag in motivation because they are common when you've been at it for that long. One day she complained about her lack of progress.

"I am so discouraged, Sue. I have been so good about what I eat and I've even started walking several miles day and the scale just won't move. What's wrong?" she asked.

I gave her my standard reply. "I need to know exactly what you are eating to determine what the problem is." And to my amazement she pulled a paper from her purse and gave it to me. It was filled out completely with portions noted as well as intake of water, milk products, and fruits and vegetables too! It was a rare sight for me to see such a complete record of someone's food intake. I was thrilled.

And Arlene's problem was evident from the first glance. It jumped right out at me that she wasn't eating enough. Yes, she was eating a beautifully balanced and nutritious diet, but there just weren't enough calories there to sustain her metabolism. I took a deep breath and dreaded having to tell her that she had to eat more.

This piece of advice never computes in the brains of people trying to lose weight. It's a recurring theme in my many years of weight loss counseling experience. Sometimes there are audible gasps of horror when I say such things to people! Their years of dieting tells them they are overweight because they eat too much and to advise them to eat more goes against everything they believe to be true.

I was pleasantly surprised when Arlene listened intently to what I was saying and agreed to follow my advice. She decided to add in another piece of fruit and perhaps a yogurt into her daily intake and she promised she'd let me know what the scale said about the changes.

When she told me the next week that she'd dropped two pounds, you've never seen two more relieved people in your life.

Starvation and deprivation is not the way to lose weight and keep it off for good. Nutritious food in normal portions will help you succeed in the weight loss game.

Things to remember from this chapter:

- Starving yourself only makes your metabolism slow down and does not result in lasting weight loss.

- As you lose weight, you need to decrease your food intake or increase your exercise.

- Excessive exercise is not necessary nor desirable.

- Lots of heavy people eat very little.

- Eat loads and loads of fruits, vegetables, whole grains, low fat dairy products, and lean meat and you will be leaner, healthier, and not hungry.

- Eat and stay satisfied. Hunger is the enemy.

Chapter 13 - Yo-Yo Dieting And The Connection To Events, Seasons, Vacations, and Holidays

There are lots of reasons that people yo-yo diet. They lose weight in anticipation of some event and then regain it after the fact. Remember Kathy from "you Gotta Have a Goal" chapter? Once her special occasion passé, her weight returned. Other people see summer fast approaching and drop the pounds. A vacation causes them to gain back everything they lost prior to the long-awaited getaway. Or all good intentions fly out of the window when a holiday pops up on the calendar.

Yo-yo dieting destroys your self-esteem over time. You develop the mindset that "I just can't do this." Well, yes you can. You proved it by succeeding in the first place.

Yo-yo dieting also destroys your metabolism. It makes losing the weight more difficult the next time you try. Please save yourself from this circle and do not allow events, seasons, vacations, or holidays to throw you off track.

Events

How many times have I seen people lose an improbable amount of weight in anticipation of an upcoming wedding? That particular goal seems to be one of the most motivating events available to dieters. I suspect it is because of the inevitable picture- taking that goes with weddings. No one wants to be preserved for posterity looking fat.

A class reunion runs a close second on the motivation scale. Seeing people from your childhood and being faced with the scrutiny of former classmates can make most people get serious about weight loss.

Yo-Yo Dieting And The Connection To Events, Seasons, Vacations, and Holidays

The question is what happens after these events? In my experience, once the huge goal has passed, the motivation wanes and folks regain the weight they have lost. It may not be an immediate response, but most people will slack off on their regimens. That is not necessarily a bad thing. The only think that makes it bad is if you totally slip back into the bad habits that got you heavy in the first place. Then the yo-yo dieting circle begins (or resumes) and everything gets more difficult.

Otherwise, reaching your goal is a huge success! Enjoy the moment! Just don't slip back into yo-yo dieting.

Diet Seasons

Weight-loss or "diet" seasons vary throughout the United States. For instance, January 15th (everyone needs two weeks to shake off the holidays) is generally the beginning of the diet season in most areas of the country because of New Year's resolutions; however, some northern parts of the country are hindered by inclement weather in the dead of winter. Their "seasons" begin in earnest in the spring when the weather moderates and people start thinking about losing layers of clothes and replacing them with bikinis.

The second busiest time of the year is September, right after school starts up again in most areas. Then mothers that were too busy to think much about themselves over the summer can reassess their goals and make their own weight and health a priority once again. Of course, the weight gained during summer vacations may also be a motivating factor.

In the very southern area of the country, diet interest is inflated in the winter months because of a huge influx of vacationers and seasonal visitors from the north. By May, many of these people migrate back to their summer homes. Some will continue with weight loss efforts when they get home; others will spend the summer months regaining the weight they lost. It's a constant yo-yo struggle for them. I'm just happy that they bother to lose the weight they gain over the summer at all. If they chose not to, and just packed on the pounds all year long, I hate to think how heavy they could become.

People who live in these southern tourist areas year-round take their vacations when the tourists leave. Their businesses are reliant on the influx of business from seasonal visitors and so when their business slows down, it's time for them to slow down, also. Routines fall by the wayside and a new relaxed atmosphere prevails.

Vacations

Many South Florida locals journey to the Bahamas by boat for the months of May, June, and July. There are many fishing tournaments held there at this time, the weather for crossing to the islands is conducive to making the trip, and it's sort of an annual pilgrimage for many of them.

What these vacations do to weight management is not a pretty sight! I've had many folks struggle (and I mean, struggle!) to lose ten pounds over the course of the winter only to regain that and more when in the islands for a few months. I'm told that the rum in the Bahamas runs a lot more often than my clients! Sweet potato fries are popular there, too. That kind of on again-off again "dieting" isn't unique to these parts, of course. It's similar to losing weight in anticipation of a cruise where the weight is regained over the course of one highly indulgent week.

One of my yo-yo dieters one day added up what she had lost as well as what she had gained. In total she had lost 33 pounds, but she had regained 17! The weight she had gained was mainly during extended vacations and celebratory trips over the course of the year.

"Just think of how thin I could be if I hadn't gone off and started fooling around during those vacations! I have to learn to be more in control while we're away," she reasoned. And she's right. That yo-yo, starve to binge behavior is not only counter-productive, it's actually harmful. It makes moderation a temporary behavior change rather than the norm.

That's not to say, however, that planned indulgences don't have a place in weight management. One of the most successful personal weight loss "runs" I've ever had was when I promised myself if I was totally "on program" for ten weeks, then I could splurge on one particular day and have whatever I wanted! Playing mind games like these with yourself can be very motivating. It's only when a seasonal pattern of weight loss and weight gain develops that I become concerned with how successful people truly are at changing their behavior to support their goals.

I've also seen people go away for weeks at a time on cruises, on vacations, even on road trips and return several pounds lighter. I always ask how they managed to lose weight on vacation and the usual response it that they devoted more time to exercise, whether it was walking on the beach or chasing grandchildren around, the extra movement more than compensated for any extra food they ate.

It's nice to see these kinds of successes because it means these people are living their lives and enjoying themselves while continuing to work towards their weight goals. You can't ask for a better success than that! Bring home a souvenir of your vacation that can grace your wall and not your hips! Extra vacation pounds are not remembrances you want to treasure.

Holidays

If vacations are one of the roadblocks to weight loss success, holidays are the openings in the asphalt into which we all sometimes fall. The problem with holidays is that they are full of family traditions that almost always revolve around food.

There's an old story that goes something like this: A man watches his wife prepare a holiday meal. She summarily cuts both ends off of the ham and then adorns it with pineapple and cloves before putting it in the pan to bake.

Her husband asks her, "Why do you cut the ends off the ham, honey?"

Without a second thought the wife responds, 'That's the way my mother always did it."

With a puzzled, "Hmmm," the husband resolves to ask his mother-in-law at the family gathering about the ham.

"Mom," he asks, "why do you always cut the ends off the ham before you bake it? I saw Lily do that and she told me she does it because that's how you taught her to cook a ham."

The mother-in-law smiles and says, "Well that's how my mother taught me."

The man then telephones his wife's grandmother and asks her, "Both your daughter and granddaughter cut the ends off of the ham before baking it because that's what you always did. Why did you do that?"

"Well son," Grandma laughs, "I don't know why they do it but I did it because I had a small pan!"

Holiday Traditions

And that's how holiday traditions involving food begin and continue.

It's the path of least resistance to mindlessly prepare the same foods in the same ways we always have for a holiday meal. In fact, there's something very comforting in doing so. It preserves memories and happiness we've enjoyed in years past. Think for a moment about the pleasure you get in making Christmas cookies with your children using the exact same cookie cutters you used with your own mother. It's that kind of nostalgia and tradition that makes holidays special and I would never suggest that you change or forego those memories. But I would suggest that you can alter the cookie recipe without damaging the tradition.

Traditional dishes generally are quite caloric. Remember that those traditional foods come from our childhoods and think for a moment about the cooking methods and nutritional criteria that existed then. Many a household used lard for their cookies and pies. Can you picture a container of bacon grease sitting on your mother's stove for use when sautéing and frying? Or am I just much older than you are? Farm families would skim the cream from the cow's milk before drinking it and guess where the cream went? Sometimes into the hand-cranked ice cream maker complete with rock salt and ice. (Am I showing my age here or what?)

My point is that times have changed, cooking methods have changed, nutritional knowledge has changed, and we all have evolved. There's no reason why we can't keep our precious food traditions and yet prepare them in a way more in keeping with our weight goals and health issues.

Keeping the flavor and lowering the calories can become a personal crusade, and by personal I mean you need not share it with anyone outside of your kitchen. Those mashed potatoes you usually make with cream and butter will taste just as good if you mash them using chicken broth and fat-free half and half. Trust me.

Likewise, an apple or pumpkin pie made with a phyllo crust will be even more beautiful a presentation than one made with the traditional pastry crust. Lower fat versions of sour cream, cheeses, and cream cheese can save your waistline while preserving your favorite holiday foods. There's even a way to make low-fat eggnog that will have you wondering why you never made it that way before. I have no substitute for the rum or bourbon, however, unless you want to really get serious and use only extract.

Of course, there are some traditional holiday recipes that simply cannot bear any tinkering in the name of healthy eating. I personally can't think of any, but if you can, you do not have to give up your favorite foods. Planning is the key to everything we do for weight loss and this situation is no different.

You can exercise a bit more to allow yourself something special. You can practice portion control and taste what you love so dearly without gorging on it. (Remember, one bite is tasting; more than that is eating!) You can alternate low and higher calorie meals or even combine low-cal foods with a richer one you simply MUST have. Moderation will allow you to enjoy yourself, preserve family traditions, and still smile when you get on the scale after the fact.

The great thing about seasons, vacations, and holidays is that you know exactly when they are happening. There's really no excuse not to plan ahead so that you can enjoy the special moments in your life.

Things to remember from this chapter:

Yo-Yo Dieting And The Connection To Events, Seasons, Vacations, and Holidays

- Let a special event be your motivator, but don't give it all up after the event is over.

- If you fall prey to this seasonal thinking, your weight loss will suffer and you will not learn to control your eating.

- A vacation does not give you license to sabotage all of your previous weight loss efforts.

- You can actually lose weight on vacation without depriving yourself of fun and food.

- Holidays present special challenges to your weight loss efforts, but you can overcome by changing the preparation of the foods you love.

- Plan ahead!

- Yo-yo dieting is terrible and it is not part of who you are today.

Chapter 14 – Measures Of Success

Success can take many different forms and it doesn't have to have anything to do with the numbers on the scale. What an alien concept!

"Hi! How are you doing?" I'll ask a client as they step towards the scale.

"Well I'll tell you after this is over." That's a favorite response. Another one is "I'll let you know in a minute," or "You tell me." All of these comments are innocent retorts to my question but there's an underlying truth to all of them.

The Power Of The Scale

The scale controls our feelings of accomplishment, our confidence, our motivation, our self-image, our moods, and our emotions. That's a lot of power to hand over to a piece of electronic machinery, don't you think? I understand totally the feeling of powerlessness before the scale, though. Having worked hard all week and deprived yourself of some terrific foods you love only to have a weight gain is a truly disheartening experience. The only way to avoid that helpless feeling is to address the measures of success we all use.

Sometimes, I just don't weigh my clients. I now know what being in a riot without riot gear feels like. Surrounded by emotional, angry, irrational dieters is not a good place to be. All that emotional response stems from there being no way to measure their success during the preceding week. Or was there a way? The answer depends on your definition of success.

Should we all really be so controlled by the numbers on the scale? Wouldn't it be better to find other ways to define our success so the counselor is not lynched when the scale isn't available? Or so we don't feel so helpless when the weight loss we expect doesn't show up exactly when we expect it to show on the scale?

Take Your Measurements

One of the very first pieces of advice I give is that dieters take their measurements on the first night of their weight loss journey and record those measurements somewhere so they are easily retrieved at a later date. Many times the scale will become stuck in one place while the weight indicated is actually shifting around on the body. This can occur when people become more active and begin to tone their muscles, although thinking you've gained several pounds of muscle after a few workouts is not realistic.

Those changing measurements give you another way to judge your success and in some cases they can be a more rewarding change than just a number on the scale. I sometimes think of people as "skinny fat" because they have no muscles tone and few curves even though they are very slender. In this case the weight is not an accurate indicator of health and fitness or possibly even a pleasing appearance. Personally, I would rather see an inch vanish from my hips or waistline than drop a few pounds on the scale.

Men, in particular, are able to judge how their measurements are changing because they usually wear a belt. Being able to see how the worn place on the belt is slowly inching its way around from your belly button to the side of your body is extremely motivating. Being able to pull a belt up "another notch" is a true success. When you have to start hand-punching new holes in your old belt you are truly on the road to goal! In any case, the measurements can help motivate you to stay with the program when you find those numbers on the scale to be immovable.

Clothing

Similarly, wearing smaller size clothing can be a real gauge of how well your efforts are paying off. Most women have several sizes of clothing in their closets. In fact, I sometimes joke that my closet used to have those rings with sizes marked on them that you find in department stores.

Fitting into a smaller size is very rewarding. It's a pleasure that you should enjoy all along your weight loss journey. It may be expensive to buy new clothes at each step of the process, but even one article of clothing in a new size can motivate you in new ways. Then feeling that article become loose will be an even greater reward. You might even find that you fit into a smaller size despite what the scale says. Many a weight loss plateau has been broken because of the realization that the scale is not indicating exactly how much you are shrinking!

Body Mass Index

Weight per se is not always an accurate indicator of success because of differences in body composition. The Body Mass Index takes into account these differences and gives us another measure of success to boot. The BMI assesses body fat using a person's height and weight, regardless of sex. The formula is:

$$BMI = Weight (lbs) \times 703 \times Height (inches)^2$$

This formula produces a number that represents percentage of body fat. A BMI between 20-25 is considered normal for most adults. As your weight decreases you will see a resulting decrease in your BMI. The health care industry will sometimes correlate BMI with various risks of disease so your health practitioner may say that your high BMI predisposes you to certain health risks like cancer or heart disease while a low BMI may predispose you to osteoporosis. Again, the BMI is not a catch-all or a cure-all but it can be another way to measure your progress.

Other Measures Of Success

First, you can understand the process and realize that if you continue to do the right things and eat the right foods you will lose weight. Period. If you don't lose, and you're being totally honest about what you're doing, talk to someone, visit the Facebook page for suggestions, or reread a section of this book.

Second, you can enjoy the changes you have made and consider each goodie passed by, and each exercise session, as a success in itself. One of the most jarring things for me is seeing people being so hard on themselves. They are their own worst enemies rather than their own best friends. It's appalling that we cannot recognize the steps we are taking to be healthier and fitter and thinner and pat ourselves on the back for each single triumph.

One particularly lovely lady has endured a year or more of true hardship and sadness, but she has continued to adhere to a healthy eating plan regardless of her personal situation. I have admired her determination, but I also now admire her spirit.

She called me not too long ago and shared a personal success story with me. It seems she had always needed her husband's help to flip her queen-sized mattress. Her husband passed away over a year ago and she just recently decided to flip that mattress herself. When I spoke to her she was so pleased with herself that she had accomplished this task on her own. It was a testament to her exercising and weight loss as well as her returning self-confidence and I was touched that she shared her story with me. I wonder what other small wonders and tiny successes other people disregard as they seek the gold ring. What a shame not to see how far you've come and congratulate yourself on making the effort.

Similar measures of success might be hauling groceries into the house without getting winded. Chasing your children or grandchildren around and enjoying the movement might signify a change that should be celebrated. Passing up dessert at your dinner out and having a pudding cup once you get home instead is a change for the better.

Thirdly, you can use your exercise regimen as a measurement of success. Exercise and activity can be very motivating when used in this way. Try tracking the minutes you exercise each day and tally them up at the end of the week. Then try to beat last week's total this week. Maybe you want to purchase a pedometer that will calculate the miles you walk each day. Then you can try to walk a little more each day of the week. Walking a little farther each day, and finally a little faster for a set distance, is a wonderful way to see how far you've come.

But don't forget the obvious successes. If you try a new activity that you have never done before, that's a wonderful accomplishment. It shows a growing confidence in your abilities that translates to success at the scale, also. Share your new experience with someone else and you might very well inspire someone else to try rollerblading or kayaking or biking, too. People tend to look at one another and think, "Well if Mary can do it then so can I." The side benefit is all that exercise and activity will show up as a lower number on the scale.

It may also show up as a lower blood pressure reading or cholesterol count or blood sugar total. The fourth and probably most important measure of your success should be your improved health. A huge weight loss is not required to improve these conditions. In my experience, and according to the medical research, a noticeable improvement in blood pressure, cholesterol, and blood sugar appears after a loss of only ten, or fifteen, or sometimes twenty pounds.

A moderate weight loss, increased activity, and an intake of healthy foods like five servings of fruits and vegetables a day may be all that's needed to allow you to stop taking medications designed to improve your health. I have seen many, many people whose doctors have happily removed them from cholesterol lowering and blood pressure medications. I tell them that it's a lot cheaper to come to eat well than it is to buy all those medications indefinitely. It's also a lot healthier! Being overweight increases the risk of other medical conditions such as certain types of cancers and gallbladder disease so you can allay these problems by losing a moderate amount of weight, too.

A moderate weight loss can also lessen the pain associated with arthritis and other joint diseases. Lessened pain usually translates to better and freer and easier movement. It can also mean sounder sleep.

Similarly, obese individuals sometimes face social ostracism, job discrimination, and lowered self-confidence simply because of their weight. While wholly unfair and sometimes denied, it's true that we are judged by our appearance. Losing excess weight can also improve these problems that are as likely to affect health and well-being as purely medical conditions.

Defining Moments In Weight Loss

So what are the "defining moments" when it is obvious that your weight loss efforts are paying off?

Among the measures of success other dieters cite are the following:

1.) Being able to go through a turnstile without turning sideways

2.) Putting on a seat belt in someone else's car without having to lengthen it

3.) Sitting comfortably in a movie theatre or airline seat

4.) Finding that your backache was because you needed to tighten up your bra because you had lost so much weight

5.) Crossing your legs

6.) Walking without your thighs brushing together

7.) Bending down to tie your shoes

8.) Cutting back on your insulin (high blood pressure meds, etc.)

9.) Being able to sit at a booth rather than a table.

and finally,

10.) A recent friend related her experience in a department store dressing room. All the cubicles were full so she slipped a pair of pants on under her skirt out in the aisle and someone yelled, "There's a size 3 out here changing in the hall!" Imagine the inward smile that outburst created!

Things to remember from this chapter:

- Don't use the numbers on the scale as your only measure of success.

- Take your measurements and refer back to them regularly.

- Know your BMI

- Understand that the health benefit of losing weight is probably the best success you can enjoy

- Celebrate the little things you do each day to move you towards your goal.

Chapter 15 – More Measures Of Success

So do you have to actually step on the scale? Yes. Yes, you do. At least, you have to at some point.

Sometimes the mere thought of weighing-in and confronting a discouraging result is enough to keep people away from the scale. The other extreme is the person who weighs themselves five times a day and panics with every movement of the numbers.

I have a relaxed attitude about weighing yourself. You are going to be discouraged if you don't see the result you want, so why not wait until you are relatively sure the numbers have gone down? I've had some people challenge me on this front, insisting that weight gains must be confronted and dealt with as soon as possible. Usually the people adhering to this philosophy are doing just fine and never have a lousy week. I can understand their viewpoint, but I also know from experience that people will abandon all weight control efforts if the scale does not reward them.

The problem is really one of perception. The scale does not necessarily accurately reflect the effort one has expended over the past seven days. There are many reasons why the scale may weigh you heavier than it should and it doesn't have anything to do with stuffing your face at the local fast food restaurant.

Weight Fluctuations

Weight loss is simply not an exact science. There are so many variables involved that it's unrealistic to expect a steady weight loss each week. Most people weigh in at a set time on a set day and I sometimes have to remind them that the fruit of all their labor during the week may not show on the scale at that exact moment. Suppose you're wearing heavier clothes than you wore last week? Suppose you ate some frozen meals that were heavy in sodium the last two days? Suppose your hormones are raging and you're retaining fluids because of it? Suppose you started a new medication that your body is trying to adapt?

Some reasons for variation in weight include:

- Weighing at different times of day. The weight difference from AM to PM can easily exceed three pounds.

- Clothing may be different. Weight measurement while wearing jeans and sweatshirts adds several pounds whereas wearing shorts and tank tops makes you instantly lighter.

- Hormones and a woman's period can add several pounds to weight one week just to have it vanish the next. It vanishes if you have denied those chocolate cravings, at least.

- Sodium. When people first start a weight loss regimen they sometimes rely on packaged meals to get them started. These meals have improved drastically in taste in the last few years but they are still high in sodium; so, while they teach what a normal portion of food looks like, they can also cause you to retain water and show as a weight gain at the scale.

- The scale itself may be malfunctioning. It is just a simple piece of machinery, after all.

- Medications can have an effect on weight, especially steroids. The weight is not fat, just water retention, but weight nonetheless.

All of these things can influence the numbers on the scale. Usually the fluctuations are water weight that should not be mistaken or confused with added body fat. Even knowing this to be true does not save us from that sinking feeling when we see the numbers on the scale going up instead of down. So what are you going to do about it?

Unfortunately, we imbue that piece of machinery, the scale, with untold measures of power over us. The numbers on the scale can either make or break our belief in ourselves, and our desire to continue to follow the healthy eating we've adopted. Should we allow it to control our actions to such a great extent?

The Scale Provides Feedback

Let me illustrate this phenomenon of scale control. Once I had a scale weighing one thing and another weighing several pounds higher. Once this news became common knowledge, everyone, and I mean everyone wanted to weigh on the lighter scale. My question to them was, "What makes you think the lighter one is accurate? Are we not looking for accuracy but just to see lower numbers on the scale?"

Guess what the answer to that one was. The whole experience showed that the numbers on the scale are absolutely the most important thing to us. It doesn't matter if it's a truth or fiction. It's what we want to see. It validates us and our weight loss efforts.

The power of the scale and the numbers over our behavior is enormous.

It takes a long time to wean people from the idea that the scale measures our self-worth. We take a weight gain as a personal affront to our dedication and perseverance when what the scale really shows is only a measure of our efforts' successfulness. The scale is just "feedback."

The scale simply tells us if what we did the previous week was effective at helping us to lose weight, or not. If we've lost weight then we can assume what we did was effective and we can continue doing what we did.

If we gain, we need to take it as ONLY feedback that our actions did not move us closer to our weight goals. The only sensible thing to do is adjust behavior and try again. Similarly, staying at the same weight means we need to tip the balance a little further in our goal direction. That might require exercising a little more or eating a little less. Determining what positive action to take after a disappointing weigh-in is what propels you forward. Fretting over it and beating yourself up for being a failure serves no purpose.

My mission is to help clients through difficult times. It is not necessarily to admonish them and highlight their mistakes. I wish I could get them to see the scale as a tool that helps move you in the right direction rather than a stumbling block.

You Must Weigh Yourself After You Lose

Weighing-in is extremely important for the people who has successfully lost weight and maintained the loss. At that point you need to set an upper limit for yourself that triggers a return to your weight loss habits. Five pounds above your goal is usually what people chose to spur them to action once again.

Still, communicating that these successful losers must weigh in each month is sometimes like talking to a wall. I believe that they know the importance of weighing in and realize that it is required of them so that they keep a close eye on their weight and lose any pounds that push them over their goal.

I don't know why people work so hard to lose weight and then let it creep back on. The only answer that seems plausible is the one mentioned previously about how people think they go "on" a diet and then go "off" a diet. But even that doesn't fully explain the total lack of responsibility for one's actions. Facing the consequences means admitting that you have gained some weight. By doing so you hopefully will get right back to your good habits and not ruin everything you have struggled for so valiantly.

Other people that avoid the scale are generally those that set their goal weights too low in the first place. Maintaining the weight loss becomes too big of a burden and they slowly regain the weight. These people should stop sabotaging themselves and simply pick another, more realistic, goal weight.

There's little in life that is more discouraging than seeing your goal weight slip away to the extreme left side of your analog scale. If that sight doesn't make you want to eat, I don't know what would! Give yourself a break and stop trying to weigh what you weighed when you got married thirty years ago, or graduated from college (or worse yet, high school), or before you had your first child. (See Chapter "You Gotta Have a Goal.") That was then and this is now and a goal weight should be one you can maintain without too much pain. It should also be one that you see each month when you weigh-in.

One of those male clients that I am so fond of came in and showed an unusual four pound gain in one month not long ago.

"Oh my," I said. "I guess you'll just have to cut back on those beers you drink while you're fishing."

With a very disgruntled look he mumbled, "Vodka and tonics." Then he turned and walked out.

The next month he was back at goal weight. Good job of using the scale as "feedback" and adjusting his behavior appropriately.

Only A Pound?

The most common outburst from people stepping on a scale is, "What?! I only lost a pound? Are these scales right? You're kidding me, aren't you?"

After all these years I cannot understand the tendency to regret losing a pound in a week. In an entire year that loss rate amounts to 52 pounds. Remember from the earlier chapter that another way of looking at it is that a pound equals 3500 calories. Losing a pound in a week means there has been a 500- calorie deficit each day during the week between the number of calories taken in and those expended. That's a lot of calories!

One pound a week is a great effort as far as I am concerned. (See "Slow and Steady Wins the Weight Loss Race.") For others it just isn't fast enough. But fast weight loss doesn't mean permanent weight loss and trying to lose too fast indicates to me that you want to get this painful experience over with as fast as you can so you can get on with your life and resume your unhealthy eating patterns. Such an attitude is not a recipe for success.

The scale is simply a feedback mechanism. If the result is not satisfactory, change something the next week and see what the result of that change is on the scale with your next weigh-in. Do not allow the scale to control your self-esteem and don't be afraid of it, either. The scale is a tool for you to use. It does not judge your actions.

Things to remember from this chapter:

- The scale does not always accurately reflect your efforts.

- The scale is just a piece of machinery to help you evaluate your efforts.

- If the result on the scale is not what you want, then do something differently the next week.

- Don't get on the scale at all if you think the result will discourage you. Just keep on keeping on.

- People at their goal weight must weigh themselves and set an upper limit to take action.

- Any weight loss is a good weight loss.

Chapter 16 – Maintaining Your Weight Loss

Maintenance involves a slowdown of your weight loss as you learn to keep it off. This time period of maintenance is the most important time in the whole process. You have to determine how much you can eat given your activity level, age, sex, and other variables and still be able to maintain the weight you've lost. Going through maintenance and continuing to try to lose weight defeats the entire purpose!

Case In Point

One gentleman worked extremely diligently to lose over thirty pounds. I was trying to teach him to maintain the loss by slowly adding more food into his diet so that he would stop losing weight and remain the same.

He bounded up to me, obviously delighted at something.

"What is it Howard?" I asked.

"Look! Just look!" he practically shouted as he more or less jumped up and down. He reminded me of a grade-school child showing his report card to his mother.

His most recent week showed a 3.6 pound weight loss. My mind worked overtime as my first thought was, "Why on earth is he losing weight on maintenance??? Is he doing the old "I don't need to learn to maintain my weight loss? I just need to lose a few more pounds-thing?" Secondly I thought, "I do not want to discourage this man as he is obviously very pleased with himself right now."

I ended up saying, "Why Howard! A three pounds plus loss! How'd you do that?"

A smile broke out over his face as he said, "I watched everything I ate this week and worked out even harder than usual."

"That's a great effort Howard, but you're supposed to be on maintenance. You aren't supposed to be losing weight on maintenance," I reminded him, all the while keeping a congratulatory smile on my face.

"Well, but I gained a pound last week."

"But that was a good thing Howard. You weren't supposed to work extra hard this week just to lose that one pound. I'm afraid you aren't learning how to maintain your loss properly if you're doing this. Do you understand the concept of 'maintenance'?"

Much to my surprise, Howard was not taken aback at all. I had expected some degree of disappointment that I questioned his success, but instead he decided to ignore me entirely. "We're going on a three month road trip vacation and I need to get down some more," he sighed.

I wanted desperately to point out that that meant he was planning to sabotage his own success by overeating with his own blessing, but I decided my words would only be wasted. The exchange serves to illustrate two major things that hinder long term weight management:

- The yo-yo nature of weight loss for many people and,

- the reticence of the majority of people to devote time and effort to learning to maintain their hard fought weight losses.

I can understand the first problem, but that second one continues to vex me. If I could only impress upon people the importance of this step in the process; for some reason I am unable, to date, to make them understand the significance of this last step.

Learning To Maintain Your Weight Is Different Than Learning To Lose It

I recently had a heated e-mail exchange with a lady who reached her goal and continued to lose weight, disregarding entirely the maintenance process. She kept trying to "get down to where she wanted to be" and found that it was too difficult and time consuming to do so. She therefore found herself overeating because of the severe deprivation she was inflicting on herself. The result was the yo-yo loss I alluded to above. She'd lose two pounds only to gain one back. Then lose 1/2 pound to gain back three. This is not maintaining your weight! This is an exercise in futility and frustration and one of the primary reasons why weight loss is often a temporary accomplishment.

For years I have counseled people and encouraged them to weigh themselves at least once a month after reaching goal. There is what I call a "mind-set" problem associated with the whole concept of weight maintenance. I encountered it last week when a woman came to me quite proud of herself for having lost around 20 pounds and ready to choose a final weight goal.

I commented, "Your weight loss has been relatively rapid. I can see where you've been working really hard at it. In fact, there hasn't been one week when you've gained!"

"Well I'd like to lose another five or six pounds, but then what happens?" she asked.

"Once you choose your final goal weight and reach that weight, you learn how to keep the weight off. We experiment with having you eat more food to see what effect it will have on your weight. We do this until we can zero in on what amount of food you can eat each day and still keep the weight off."

"You mean I have to eat more?" she asked with a look of total dismay.

"Well of course you have to eat more. You don't want to be losing any more weight. You want to stay the same now and halt the loss, right?"

"But if I eat more I'll gain the weight back," she whined.

"No, if you eat too much you'll gain the weight back. If you eat just enough it will simply stop the loss and keep you where you are," I assured her.

She shot me a look of total panic as she said, "But you've got me programmed to lose weight and now you want me to eat more. I don't get it."

This is where I took on the most consoling and soothing voice I could muster. "You have to change your mind-set from losing to keeping it off. It's not an easy thing to shift gears like that but it's something you must do. You cannot learn maintenance by trying to lose weight while you are doing it. You have to be satisfied with your weight loss and absolutely want to remain at your goal weight. Losing weight and maintaining weight loss are two separate skills."

Do The Math Again

Most people reach their goal weight without ever bothering to "do the math" once they reach goal. They never discover exactly what they can eat at and still stay the same weight. Maintenance requires that you stabilize your weight, but in a structured way.

A hit or miss method of eating this and that does not give you the information you need to keep the weight off.

This type of behavior stems from an over-confidence that can ultimately lead to weight gain. Maintenance cannot be based on confidence and self-esteem, two variable components in our lives that shift and change depending on circumstances.

Maintenance must be based on a solid, non-emotional accounting method. Thinking you are "finished" your diet is a popular notion once you reach your goal weight. Thinking that you must continue to monitor your food intake is not popular, despite supporting evidence that this is the only substantiated way to maintain a loss.

There must be a reason that this concept is so unacceptable to most people. I go through this same spiel over and over again. The results are sometimes wonderful but equally as often they are disastrous. Someone will work and strive to lose weight and then blow off the maintenance aspect and end up regaining all they lost. Not only is it a waste of effort, I personally think it's a blow to anyone's self-esteem to lose weight and regain it like that. Yo-yo dieting may also serve to undermine your efforts by dropping your metabolism in the long run.

Without learning how much food you can eat and still keep the weight off, you are doomed to a life of constant dieting. You overeat and gain the weight and then diet to lose it. Wouldn't it be better, easier, and less stressful just to maintain the status quo and keep the weight off for good? Couldn't you them devote the time and energy you give to dieting to a better cause?

I have begun to introduce this concept to people far in advance of them reaching their goal weights in an effort to further incorporate the maintenance concept into their expectations. I lecture them and probably repeat myself too much about the importance of thinking of weight loss as a two-part process: lose and maintain.

Celebrate Yourself, Every Day

Another mental problem with maintaining a weight loss is the lack of celebration associated with "staying the same." While losing weight, people are constantly rewarded and their success celebrated. Inside the group they are congratulated, and their efforts encouraged. Outside the group they are being complimented on their new shape, appearance, perhaps even their physical fitness.

Now suppose you lost 45 pounds ten years ago. Where is all that positive reinforcement now? People no longer congratulate you on your appearance because to them, that's simply how you are supposed to look. It's hard to use physical fitness as a milestone because you have been exercising for so long it is difficult to find a new challenge.

Since there's no specific number attached to maintaining your loss, like losing 10 pounds for example, you can't blow your own horn. And yet, people maintaining their weight loss are working just as hard to keep the weight off as people trying to lose it in the first place.

I mentioned to one notable "loser" who takes untold pleasure in compliments and outside reinforcement that she should steel herself for the day the compliments end. I suggested that three years down the road she would not be enjoying all the attention she is getting right now. Already new people she meets do not recognize her accomplishment simply because they never knew her when she was overweight. Sometime soon everyone will just expect her to be her current weight. They will not acknowledge her loss nor reward her with compliments.

Several days after our conversation she said, "You told me compliments would stop but THEY HAVEN'T. I saw neighbors from out of the country that hadn't seen me for a year and they were amazed at how different I look."

166

Naturally, I responded with, "That's great! Doesn't that make you feel good?" But what I was thinking was, "I didn't tell you the compliments would stop to burst your bubble or spoil your fun. I told you that to prepare you for the inevitable time when your motivation to keep the weight off has to come from inside yourself rather than from other people."

She did, however, take my comments to heart because she had a unique way of celebrating her one- year anniversary of her weight loss. At the one-year mark she took a digital photo of herself and sent it out to distant family, friends, and old neighbors. These people had no idea she was embarking on a weight loss program and so were extremely excited and supportive of her new appearance. She told me that the comments and notes she received were a "real shot in the arm" at a time of waning enthusiasm on her part.

Revealing her success to a select group of people at a later date served her well. Their responses encouraged her to stay the course. I worry about her lack of internal motivation and her reliance on the acceptance of others. On the other hand, maybe you can use her tactic of before and after photos to regenerate your own enthusiasm for your efforts.

Being fit and trim and healthy is certainly its own reward, and being able to fit into whatever article of clothing you wish to wear is a true success. Still, it would be nice to receive some accolades for all the effort expended. As a successful maintainer myself, I understand that it is difficult to remain motivated solely by your own resources. I suggest you reward yourself with monthly or bi-monthly treats. A special mani/pedi for the ladies maybe, and a massage for the gentlemen. Anything that celebrates your achievement will help keep you motivated.

Stop Losing When You Reach Your Goal

There is yet another pitfall of keeping the weight off for good that strikes the very lucky individual, usually a younger man or woman who stays very active. In this case, the person will go on maintenance, begin eating more food, and continue to lose more weight. I know we all wish we had this kind of problem, but it truly is a problem for the person experiencing it. Some people can lose an additional ten pounds and end up well below their goal weight. The extra loss can sometimes put people in an unhealthy underweight range.

The solution to this problem seems simple enough. Just eat more! But it isn't easy to convince someone who has limited their food intake for an extended period of time to reach their goal weight to eat more. They simply do not want to risk their success by eating more food. Unfortunately, the easy loser needs to do just that. They need to eat enough to stop their weight loss and they may find that they can eat much more than they used to.

Surprise! You Can Eat More Than You Thought!

This pleasant surprise usually occurs because increased exercise has resulted in increased muscle mass which has resulted in a higher metabolism. Believe me when I tell you that this is the best possible scenario for anyone that struggles with their weight. I encourage these lucky folks to enjoy their success. Don't overdo, but do track your intake, see how much food you can eat at given this time and circumstance, and then eat a healthy diet of nutritious foods.

One particular lady pops to mind. She struggled to get to goal and she fought for each pound she lost. She worked out, she ate a limited amount, she agonized (and I mean, agonized) over why she couldn't lose the last few pounds. Finally we raised her goal weight when I convinced her that the struggle to get to the magic number she had in mind was just too difficult.

She went on maintenance, began eating more, and those few pounds she had tried so hard to lose just magically disappeared. I was, of course, concerned with that outcome since her weight was supposed to stabilize on maintenance but she had really been doing maintenance for weeks when she was trying unsuccessfully to lose the last few pounds. We decided that the extra food intake actually increased her metabolism just enough to get her to her original goal. Both of us were pleasantly surprised. Actually, that's an understatement. I think she was overjoyed!

It became obvious that she had not been eating enough to stoke her metabolism, an issue we revisited over the course of her weight loss. I always had to make sure she was eating enough. Finally, in maintenance she found she could eat more than she thought and still be at her goal weight. Last I heard she was happily enjoying a few glasses of wine over the course of a week and eating the foods she loved. She always enjoyed meats and cheese over sweets and continued to enjoy them at her lower weight. The point to learn is that it is not always necessary, nor advisable, to give up the foods you love in order to see the scale move.

Maintaining your hard fought weight loss is a very individualized process, as these examples illustrate. Many times maintenance is the time when you learn the little idiosyncrasies about your own body's way of using food and calories. Variables come into play that you may not have considered to be important over the course of your weight loss.

If you approach this period as a detective might: watching for results of actions, adjusting behavior accordingly, slowly add healthy food items into your diet, and always recording your food intake, you will remove the emotional component and rely instead on the rational approach. The rational approach always makes the process easier and more likely to bring on long- term weight loss success.

Maintaining is a period when you have to be diligent about writing down everything you eat, in what portions, and weighing yourself regularly. If you continue to lose weight, you eat a little more the next week. If you gain weight, you eat a little less. If you stay the same weight, then add in a little bit more food and see if you gain or not. It's easy. Trial and error will stabilize your weight and give you the information you need to maintain your weight loss.

Things to remember from this chapter:

- You have to learn to maintain your weight loss in a structured way.

- Losing weight and maintaining the loss are two different and separate skills.

- Without learning your unique maintenance strategy, you are doomed to a life of yo-yo dieting. You deserve so much better,

- Find ways to celebrate your success at maintaining your weight loss.

Chapter 17 – The Importance Of Group Support

The importance of group support cannot be underestimated in its ability to inspire, motivate, and encourage behavior modification. This is the reason for the Facebook group page which supports the readers of Win When You Lose. Visit at http://www.facebook.com/WinWhenYouLose. There is always comment and discussion among a variety of divergent people in terms of their culture, geography, occupation, and social background. Despite the differences among all these people, they are actually more alike than they are dissimilar.

Our Weight Issues Bring Us Together

The common fight against the tendency to overeat and the so-called "battle of the bulge" bridges any gap in other areas of their lives. They openly share their experiences and tips to stay on a healthy eating program and bring many different tactics and strategies to share with one another.

As such, they relate to one another on a personal level. Their sharing of triumphs and tragedies occurs because they feel a close bond with one another. Being comfortable with people in the group brings a deeper level of self-disclosure and comment.

When you are comfortable within a support group is when every topic is fair game. It's when you can really get at the deeper emotional issues involved in overeating because the group participants are more open and honest within a group where they feel safe. Revealing innermost fears and dreams is a difficult thing to do in a group setting, but these friends all know they are sharing the same condition and there is nothing anyone can say that someone else hasn't experienced.

Words Of Wisdom From The Group

This shared commonality between group participants is more important than you might imagine. When I was losing my weight, I had reached a plateau of several weeks and was thoroughly discouraged. During a weekend phone call with a family member, I expressed my feelings. Now, this person has always been overweight but at that time he was making a concerted effort, aided by diet drugs and exercise, to trim down. I felt we had a common concern and I felt safe in turning to him for help and guidance.

"I just don't know what's going on," I lamented. "I'm not eating much. I'm exercising. I'm doing all the things I've been doing up to this point and I just can't lose any more weight."

"Well, I guess you'll just stay fat then," he responded.

I didn't let on that I was upset but when I hung up that phone I burst into tears. I was just crushed.

Sharing this episode several days later, I expressed my discouragement.

One very smart lady asked me, "Sue, would you ask your relative for a million dollars?"

"Of course not!"

"Well why not?"

"Because he doesn't have it," I answered.

"Exactly," she said. "You can't expect anyone to give you what they don't have. He didn't have the encouragement and solace to give to you. It doesn't matter why he didn't have it to give to you, does it? The fact is you looked in the wrong place for something you needed."

Seek Out People Who Will Support You Best

From that moment on I went to people I knew would be supportive and understanding. I have to admit that my husband has always been my biggest supporter, but not all dieters have the luxury of family support. Always bring your problems, troubles, desires, and needs to the group and I guarantee you will find a listening ear to hear you and a soft shoulder to lean on. The best support is the support of those people who have been and are going through the exact same experiences that you are, be they good or bad. Just always expect honesty because you are likely to get it.

I try to take the lead in being as honest and open as possible. I believe in sharing both the times I've overcome an obstacle to weight loss as well as sharing the times I've failed. No one is perfect and everyone needs to recognize that there will be times and circumstances when you need help.

Among the information shared in a group are: recipe ideas, cooking techniques, tips on what products are most useful (and usually where to buy them for the least amount of money), how and where to eat out and stay within the limits of the plan, what to do when company arrives and shakes your whole routine to its very foundation,, what to do when you "fall off the wagon" and how to get back on, how emotional eating can be overcome, how to deal with people who would rather you didn't succeed (saboteurs), how to enlist the aid of your family and friends, staying motivated, exercise and activity , and stories of successes and not-so-successful experiences.

Many people shy away from the group experience and it's always to their own detriment. I cannot express adequately the importance of the group. There is no doubt whatsoever in my experience that people without social support generally fail miserably. "Going it alone" is really a recipe for disaster.

Going It Alone Is Too Hard

I can think of many, many people who have insisted that they want to "try it on my own." It doesn't take long before I see them again, tens of pounds heavier than when I saw them last. Naturally, gaining back the weight then makes it even more difficult for them to admit defeat and try again. The question then becomes: What alternative do you have? You can continue to eat and feel lousy about yourself. Then you'll get heavier and be even unhappier. Or you can swallow your pride and get the help you need to be successful. Unfortunately, no one else can make that decision for you.

Behavior modification like that needed to lose weight and keep it off must be supported through a group experience. You can feel uncomfortable sharing your feelings with others and that's certainly OK, but please, at least visit the Facebook group. You will absorb much information and motivation by just being there. You don't have to even participate if you don't want to.

Men tell me they don't like to share with a group but I have to tell you that men are vocal and funny and insightful. There just need to be more of them. Without generalizing too much, I have to say most men think they don't need help, they can "fix it" on their own, and they do not enjoy the sharing aspect of groups. They also tend to believe if they don't eat all day until dinner, the weight will fall off. They seem to do all right with the presentation of nutritional information, but when it comes down to the innermost reasons we overeat, most men become uncomfortable.

Unfortunately, confronting those demons is the only way to succeed in keeping the weight off. Men, more so than women, think of restricted eating as a "diet," a temporary change necessary to reach a desired goal. They can control their overeating for a time to succeed in reaching their goal (men seem extremely goal oriented), but then their bad habits return and so does the weight.

Take Inspiration From Those Who Have Succeeded

Successful dieters are the best resource for inspiration for the group. These are the people who know what it takes to win the weight war. They are tangible evidence that everyone can reach their goal weight and stay there for the long haul. They are a rich resource of information and inspiration that is sometimes neglected, so please, please offer your wisdom to the group. We need you! Your experiences are common to everyone. Relating those experiences makes other people feel less alone and more like part of the group.

There's almost a level of "payback" involved. Successful "losers" are expected to share their experiences with others on a regular basis since they reaped the rewards of the group experience during their weight loss. This payback, pay forward, aspect is sometimes overlooked. I hope you feel a duty and responsibility to help the group succeed.

You get what you give. At any given time, in any given support group, there are givers and takers. The givers are the ones losing weight and feeling good about themselves. They give the rest of the group inspiration and determination. The takers are the ones that are struggling at that particular moment. They need the support, the encouragement, and they need to see others succeed to know they can do it themselves.

This give and take is what makes group support so valuable. If you have a challenge confronting you, pose the issue to the group. I guarantee someone in the group has met and overcome the very same challenge. Likewise, if you have succumbed to temptation, let the group help you get back on track. Surely someone else there had the identical situation arise in their own lives. These changing roles are what keep the group dynamics working. Your participation, whatever your role, is vital to the success of the group.

The Safety Net Of The Group

At a motivational seminar many years ago, the speaker tossed a ball of yard into the air and when someone spoke she held the end of the yarn and tossed the ball to the person speaking. When the next person spoke, the person with the yarn held the end and tossed the ball to the next speaker. In this way, and with a room of talkative people, the yarn soon formed a mesh pattern.

It was an interesting exercise because we mentioned how the group interaction actually wove a "safety net" to keep people from falling, faltering, or failing. It also illustrated that the strength of the group is in the interaction between the participants. Since that is true, it is also true that any supportive group can provide the "safety net." The only requirement is that the group be willing to talk about their experiences, share their coping strategies, and be fighting the same demons. The support network therefore succeeds for Overeaters Anonymous, AA, NA, Weight Watchers, various illness support groups, community associations, and other places where people have common ground for discussion. One should assume that the group support works to help people meet their goals or else the structure would not be so pervasive.

Buddy Up

Losing weight can sometimes be a singularly solitary endeavor. I know because my husband can eat whatever he wants whenever he wants and will always weigh less than I do! Therefore, keeping to my exercise and eating plan is oftentimes a lonely experience. I feel less isolated being with a group of people who share my problems and challenges. It makes the struggle easier. And less isolated and easier usually translates to more successful.

Not every group will give you the feeling of belonging. That feeling is one that needs cultivation. Pairing people or establishing a buddy-relationship with another group participant facilitates a sense of belonging among the participants. Don't hesitate to approach a Facebook group member directly to establish that one-on-one connection.

The group experience far exceeds just a social gathering. Still, the social aspect of the group cannot be ignored. I once asked a very quiet group participant what she got from the group.

"I live alone and this group is the most interaction I have in my whole week. I learn a lot from everyone and I'll lose weight when I put my mind to it. Don't you worry, honey, I'm doing just fine," she told me.

And I didn't worry about her again. I simply realized that we were fulfilling a need for her. It may not have been the service I had in mind, but it was valuable service nonetheless.

Help one another. It will make you stronger to do so.

Things to remember from this chapter:

- Group support is a valuable resource when you are trying to lose weight.

- The Facebook "Win When You Lose" page is there for you all. Please participate! I will be monitoring it and interjecting thoughts form time to time. You can also visit the website/blog at http://www.winwhenyoulose.wordpress.com.

- Think about finding a weight loss buddy for a one-on-one relationship

- Successful dieters are important contributors. We need you!

- Remember the "safety net" of group interaction. It is available to you.

Facebook Page For You

The supporting Facebook page at Win When You Lose is for you, the readers. It is a safe forum for discussion and interaction. I will be posting recipes, notes of encouragement, and links to informational material on a regular basis. Please join the Win When You Lose community and make your weight loss dreams come true.

Chapter 18 – Believe Me, I Understand

Of those readers mentioned in the Introduction, the very overweight person, the person who needs to lose twenty pounds, the person whose metabolism drops with age, the one who gains weight during menopause, and the one with four sizes of clothes in their closet, I fall into several categories. Over time, I have fallen into all these categories.

My weight problems have haunted me my entire life and I have no doubt that they will always plague me. I simply cannot eat what I want, when I want, and maintain a healthy weight. Some of the blame for the situation rests with my family's genes. Both my mother and father's siblings, that I can recall, were all overweight. There's definitely a family heritage of large butts and broad hips on both sides of my family tree.

Mom – My First Glimpse

My mother fought the tendency to be overweight tooth and nail. I can see her eating cottage cheese and fruit for dinner while my father and a much younger me ate steaks and French Fries. I can see her lying on the floor trying to do the exercises she had ripped out of women's magazines.

One particularly memorable day I came home from school and found her sitting on the floor with her legs outstretched in front of her. She would rise up on one cheek, thrust the other leg and cheek forward, and thus scoot across the floor, alternating legs.

"Hey Mom," I said. "What's that one supposed to do?"

I got down on the floor with her and tried it myself. It was pretty taxing and it took a fair bit of coordination. It also provoked serious rug burn.

Huffing and puffing she replied, "It's supposed to get rid of the fat on my butt, that's what!"

I'm not sure why that picture of her remained so vivid to me over the years but it always makes me smile. The lady tried to keep things under control. She just didn't realize that the only thing that will remove the McDaniel love handles is liposuction, something that had yet to be invented at the time.

I can see her cinching in her small waist and patting her stomach with her hand, bemoaning the fact that she could never diet away her stomach. In those days she would shimmy into a girdle (no Spanx yet) and, in retrospect, look fabulous. Unfortunately, she died much too early and I never got to tell her how, as I aged, I came to understand her struggle in a very personal way.

Psychologists in the popular press recently criticized such mothers. Supposedly their efforts to keep their weight under control and retain their figures generated negative self-images within my own generation. Similarly, mothers today are discouraged from imposing "negative self-images" on their current children.

The problem with these arguments is that there is a definite difference between self-image and body-image. Confusing the two is where children can be harmed. My mother always told me that I could be or do whatever I wanted. She encouraged me to be strong and assertive. That reinforced a positive self-image. She did, however, recognize that both of us needed to work on our weight control and nutrition. She, therefore, attempted to influence and help improve my body- image. I don't believe that she ever confused the two separate issues so I don't normally confuse them either.

Parents

Today's parents must educate their children about nutrition, health, and exercise. The education can't come from derision or criticism, but rather should be from example. Parents that work at nutrition and exercise are beneficial role models. Most of them intuitively recognize the difference between self- and body- image and do not equate the two in dealings with their own children. Admittedly, you can overdo a good thing and be obsessively concerned with weight and body image to the point of detriment. Sometimes children need to be made aware of the fact their bodies do not determine their self-worth, especially if they are being ridiculed and teased at school. But in most cases, showing your children that you consider it important to be health and body conscious is a good thing.

Parents have a great deal of control over their children's eating patterns. Whoever buys the food and prepares the meals can introduce healthy eating patterns as a normal part of family life. No food should ever be forbidden unless health reasons demand it; even for someone trying to lose weight, no food is off limits. Influencing your family's perception of healthy portions and advocating good nutrition and exercise are not efforts that should be faulted.

The body is the window to the soul and caring for that precious vessel is what allows us to do good works and pursue our dreams. Granted, the media portrayal of the "perfect" body is far from perfect. I cringe when I see ultra-thin models in magazines geared to young women just as I wonder what message young men get when they see male models with pec implants.

Those unrealistic expectations, however, cannot be pinned on mothers or fathers who valiantly fight the battle of the bulge. If I myself did not reign in my impulses, I'd easily balloon to 300 pounds without blinking. How healthy would that be? Better to make the effort, don't you think? And as for our children, if we ourselves endured a childhood of ridicule based on our weight, our desire is generally to save them from whatever pain we suffered.

Childhood

As a child, I had to shop at the Lane Bryant store. No offense meant to Lane Bryant, of course, it's just that having those labels rub up against your neck day in and day out was not only embarrassing, it was a constant reminder that you were different from everyone else. You were different in a big way. I longed to shop in the regular stores where the cute little girls with the sparkly hair ribbons shopped.

I can remember the dreaded "before school starts" shopping trip. I was always in the "chubby" section while I'm sure my male counterparts were in the "husky" areas. How awful for impressionable children to endure such name-calling, from marketers, of all people.

One particular year, fifth grade, perhaps, I recall trying on a hideous green and red plaid dress with a white Peter Pan collar. I looked like an obese bagpipe player. I stood under the lights on a circular platform for my mother to inspect me. This wasn't done in the fitting room, but rather out in the showroom where the entire store could see you.

"Turn around, Susie," she said.

I turned, praying that she wouldn't like that dress.

"It looks beautiful, honey," she cooed. "We'll take it."

"But MOM," I moaned.

Forty-five years later I still hate that dress.

Of my own weight problems, I vividly remember elementary school gym class. The gym teacher, who I talk about later in this book, degraded and ridiculed me beyond all good reason. His example set the stage for like treatment from my classmates. I was forever the brunt of jokes, and always picked last for every sports team. Not that that is unusual. Most people say the same thing and I sometimes have to wonder who was picked at other times if we were all chosen last? Playing softball over the summer during my final year between elementary and junior high school helped me gain back some confidence and self-esteem, setting the stage for an easy transition to middle school.

Weight was, of course, a constant war for me. I became determined to lose weight when my family moved from one location to another between eighth and ninth grades. I realized that move was an opportunity to shed the old me that everyone thought they knew and reinvent myself. I entered ninth grade with a svelte new figure thanks to limiting my food intake over the summer. I enjoyed that year of school with the abandon of a young child. I was suddenly a social butterfly, all because I had lost weight. It became obvious to me then that weight is an extremely limiting issue. It holds you down and restricts your life more than you can know.

Later

Subsequent years saw me dieting down to the lowest I've ever weighed for my wedding. Then I got pregnant and thanked my son day in and day out for the opportunity to indulge every food desire I had squelched for so many years. I fell in love with peanut butter, Twinkies, and Big Macs. I ballooned to 200 pounds by the time I went into labor.

Five months later we went to the beach with friends. They wanted us to drink and party and we declined.

One friend looked at me and said, "Oh, I get it. You're pregnant again."

Believe Me, I Understand

I wasn't.

Once again the dieting started and I regained some semblance of control over my eating. Though difficult and depriving, the control felt good. I never got as thin as I had been prior to the pregnancy, but it was an acceptable weight.....until I unexpectedly lost my father. I wallowed in sadness and ate to dull the pain.

After that I found myself at a national weight loss chain. A neighbor had suggested it to me a year earlier and I had taken great offense. Now I thank her for her insight and concern. Learning how to eat healthfully was a great awakening for me. In fact, it became the basis of a lifelong calling to help others achieve their weight loss goals. And I lost 47 pounds, too.

Now, over twenty years later, with minor ups and downs, I am still maintaining a healthy weight. I went on to become a group motivational speaker for the next twelve years, followed by years of weight loss coaching for individuals. Hopefully this book will extend my reach and allow me to encourage more people to control their weight and control their lives.

Please believe me when I tell you can do anything you want to do. You can lose the weight, you can reinvent yourself, you can be who you want to be, go where you want to go, and accomplish whatever you desire. Do not let anyone tell you otherwise.

Chapter 19 – Thank You So Much

I thank you all very much for the opportunity to share what I have learned about weight loss with you in this book. Your success is my success and I would love to hear about your experiences. Please feel free to contact me at the Win When You Lose blog (http://www.winwhenyoulose.wordpress.com/). You can also visit me and other readers on Facebook, at http://www.facebook.com/WinWhenYouLose. A future YouTube channel will be added with demonstrations and videos to complement the Win When You Lose book. It will be announced on both the above Facebook page and on the blog.

As a very special friend once said, "Thank you all for a really nice time".

Susan

For further information on the National Weight Control Registry you can visit their website at http://www.nwcr.ws . If you are over age 18, have lost thirty pounds or more, and maintained the loss for at least one year, they would love to have you participate in their study. The registry was established in 1994 by Rena Wing, Ph.D. and James O. Hill, Ph.D. Only one in six overweight or obese Americans lose weight and maintain the loss. Research into long-term weight loss management is important for all of us.

www.ingramcontent.com/pod-product-compliance
Lightning Source LLC
Chambersburg PA
CBHW070648290526
45790CB00001B/234